CONTENTS

Introduction

Limerence is, quite frankly, unrequited or impossible love gone wrong. It is the tendency to 'fall for' specific characters who resonate with you uniquely, in an *implausibly* intense, agonising way. In a way that pushes you into a **chronic state of addiction** – in a way that allows these individuals to have far more of an emotional hold over you than *any* human being should ever have. And goodness, the emotions that limerence evokes in you in response to these people's treatment of you are wild. Seemingly entirely distanced from your former self's rationality, you will be carried to the peaks of euphoria, only to subsequently be pushed off the edge of a precipice and <u>freefall towards abject depression</u>. Over and over again.

It goes without saying that there is no psychological condition quite like limerence. It is such a fascinating, all-consuming, surreal phenomenon that it is easy to dissolve into it and let your identity slip away. Despite desperately craving freedom from the emotional rollercoaster, you find yourself incapable of imagining your life untinged by the bittersweet euphoria that is so intrinsic to the state. The peaks and troughs of the limerent experience could not be more different, but they go hand in hand. They are two opposite poles of the same thing: passion that has gone *way too far*. An addiction that you should never have fallen prisoner to in the first place.

I have risen to the challenge of writing a book whose contents will render you completely immune to limerence, *without* you needing to suppress any aspects of your personality or kiss goodbye to **enlivening, exciting emotions** in general. Being a neuroscientist and a natural empath, I find it rewarding beyond belief to present the basis of limerence from a multidisciplinary standpoint and impart every last truth about human relationship dynamics that I have collected over the years to struggling limerents. After all, my life used to be profusely and absurdly dominated by this aberrant form of love; those of you who are familiar with my online content will know that I spent years of my life psychologically and physiologically controlled by limerence, in a state of agony, learned helplessness and devastating existentialism.

Fortunately, limerence never disturbed my academic life, because my inherent perfectionism and drive for success allowed autopilot to take over. The emotional chaos I endured did, however, bleed into every other realm of my human existence, until I learnt how to break free a decade ago and slingshot myself towards an entirely new reality.

Many psychiatrists attempt to treat small fragments of the limerence symptomatology, mildly alleviating your pain but falling short at targeting the root cause and correcting it. The nuance is that limerence, being a form of pathological love, *cannot be* correctly conceptualised when its symptoms are considered individually; reductionism is flawed when it comes to treating such conditions. Nor can you treat the fundamental issues aligning you with limerence through attempting *to blunt the pain* it puts you through with antidepressants or alcohol. Whilst therapy at least attempts to tackle the underlying drivers of limerence, most therapists fail to *correctly* identify, isolate and rigorously treat them because they are unfamiliar with the reality of enduring the condition – they don't quite know *what* underpins it, or comprehend that such a degree of person addiction is even possible. Thus, they are equally unable to catalyse lasting change in you.

In this book, we are going to cover limerence exhaustively, first methodically working through its biological and psychological underpinnings to provide you with a crystal clear understanding of what it actually is/represents. Then, we will learn how to truly cure it (once and for all) from a multidisciplinary and well-rounded, but above all, *human,* standpoint. When you finish reading, you will comprehend precisely what this behavioural pattern is, why *you* have aligned with it, and exactly what you need to do to transform your thoughts, emotions, attachment style and demeanour towards life in such a way that you are **still yourself**, but **permanently *limerence-immune***.

1. If You Want to Recover, You Will

Whether you have only known life with limerence as a prominent component or you have recently fallen into your first limerent episode, you must realise that you are not the passive receiver of these feelings. We tend to think of ourselves as little worms in the earth, incapable of predicting who or what is going to impinge on our mental health. I want you to shatter this paradigm, for it promotes falsehoods and does not serve you in any way. Your limerent object (LO) is only capable of unlocking this cocaine-like euphoria, consequent grief and abnormal obsession in you because their personality, energy and treatment of you all complement your unhealed wounds and unmet needs; the root cause of your feelings is you, and we need to change your inner wirings so that you are no longer a psychological fit for limerence.

Only by truly understanding the basis of limerence from neuroscientific, psychological, and spiritual perspectives can you rewire your subconscious mind away from the allure of this tenacious addiction. In this book, I shall teach you how to do this and demonstrate to you that you can leave limerence behind and become completely, one hundred percent immune – for life. If you assimilate this information and commit to actively recovering, your life will never be the same; you will look back in a few years and wonder, amused and bewildered, how another person was *ever* capable of inspiring such mania and depression in you. I know that this outcome will seem like a pipe dream in your current state, but it is an absolute promise.

2. Is It Necessary to Live a Dull, Purposeful, Stoic Existence?

Most of the limerence-related material you will come across tries to warm you up to the idea that you, as someone prone to this obsessional state, will constantly be fighting a battle. That you *either* get to experience a rich emotional life and suffer from limerence, OR you commit to being 'sensible' and forgo intensity completely, settling for dull connections void of 'magic'.

Since you will be aware that limerence is far more devastating and embarrassing than it is exciting, you may have even come to terms with this supposedly necessary compromise of '**living while avoiding highs**'. At this point, you're probably willing to do anything to shield yourself from the horrors of the limerent crashes. However, another part of you will be voicing itself in equal strength, imploring you to remember that being limerent has also gained you access to a psychedelic, childhood-reminiscent spectrum of emotions. Would life not be meaningless without butterflies, spontaneity, uncertainty and being pushed outside your comfort zone by interesting individuals?

Worry not, for I have fantastic news for you. Adhering to stoicism and renouncing all highs will be <u>entirely unnecessary</u> once you succeed in transforming your self-concept in the ways that I will describe in detail in upcoming chapters. Ultimately, I do not want you to have to 'resist' the temptation of limerence, because that does not constitute recovery; I want you to become **a version of yourself that cannot become limerent**, and hence, does not miss or even think about limerent highs. Consequently, there is precisely zero need to fret about the possibility that life will be colourless when your days are no longer controlled by LOs. In Chapter 32, you will also learn how to use your quirky, astute limerent mentality to your advantage.

Yes, not only are you going to break free from the nightmare that is limerence, but you are also going to learn how to capitalise on that incandescent energy and passion that is currently only being directed towards **the fantasy bond** between you and your LO. Right now, you are not acquainted with this limerence-immune version of yourself, so you cannot imagine a life <u>without a LO at its centre</u> being sufficiently interesting, but I can promise you that this is an illusion that is part of the evolutionary blueprint of limerence – part of how these pathological, horrible feelings are *designed* to hijack your brain.

Once you learn to intercept the driving causes of limerence and alter your belief systems, no other human will even be *able* to offer you the initial dopamine 'glimmer' that leads to limerence. You will remain your lively, passionate, curious self, but will no longer suffer from life chapters dominated by limerent episodes. I have been completely limerence-free for nearly a decade, and can truly say that my life is still thrilling and euphoric, but just in different, *truly* rewarding ways that do not come back to sabotage me.

3. Stoicism Is Only A Temporary Fix

The conventional mantra that you must 'learn to live with your yearning for your LO', and live purposefully regardless of your pain, does serve <u>one purpose</u>. That purpose is only in helping you exit the current state that you are in; I must concede that initially you *will* need to actively resist the urge to self-soothe by seeking your LOs attention. If you are reading this and are currently limerent, I do want you to realise that you will have to spend a period of a few weeks 'forcing' yourself to live with intention – forcing yourself to gain positive momentum. This will involve you ignoring your LO (or, if you cannot cut contact, ensuring that you do not engage in deep conversations with them that trigger you), as well as avoiding exacerbating your pain by ditching all music/ media that transmits themes of **overbearing, painful love**. This initial, stoic stage of recovery will also require that you force yourself to see your friends and family (even when you feel blue and only want a 'hit' from your LO), exercise, eat a healthy, nourishing diet, and finish work that may not feel like your priority.

By going cold turkey in this way (i.e. 'forcing' yourself *away from* indulging fantasies about your LO/interacting with them in 'that specific way' that you love while focusing *as intently as you can* on other things), you will detach from this particular LO and move on with your life. There is no way around this initial stage of intentional detachment. Your brain wants to keep you a prisoner in the limerence chamber, sustained by its misguided belief that you are going to reproduce with this individual and perpetuate the human species if it rewards you with dopamine upon you *attempting to get closer to them*. If this was not laughable enough in itself (since we all know that limerence, by nature, entails either unrequited love or impossible love), these same evolutionary mechanisms will be activated identically if you are intoxicated by someone of the same gender.

The brain regions implicated in limerence do not care if a). your LO is a). someone of the opposite gender who you have had a real fling with or if b). you identify as gay and are obsessing over someone you chat to on Twitter but who lives across the world. Evolution prioritises pair-bonding and reproduction over everything, with behaviours related to it only potentially rivalled by those that promote food-seeking (hence why obesity and food addiction can be as problematic for some people as limerence). Therefore, despite our real strategy being to inoculate you against limerence and allow you to 'reality-flip' into a new life where LOs do not even exist, we must *temporarily* learn to sit with and accept pain; when you pull your brain's little grubby fingers away from the cookie jar, best believe s/he will kick up a fuss.

A great way to look at this cold turkey transition is to remember that limerence, by its very nature, always subjects you to excruciating, **white-hot emotional pain** (as well as many more collateral emotions like guilt, humiliation, anger). Limerence is invariably a horrifically painful experience, and often unpredictably so. Over the course of a single limerent episode, you are guaranteed to <u>find yourself emotionally floored</u> when you least expect it. Often, this will be due to **your LO's behaviour** and your conclusions about it: a single look of disdain from them may send you running to a restaurant bathroom to cry before a meeting, and seeing an unexpected social media upload from them celebrating their partner's achievements will be sure to make you *severely depressive* right before a family reunion. Just as frequently, however, you will cycle through states of misery triggered by **nothing but your own thoughts**, e.g. suddenly remembering that they said that they'd be on holiday this weekend (and picturing them making memories), or even just randomly lamenting the fact that you two are not together. Limerence will serve you up at least a jolt of agony a day, which you will typically experience in highly poignant, personal ways.

Therefore, the initial discomfort (and, at times, grief) that accompanies the <u>earliest stage</u> of recovery is nothing to worry about. You are more than capable of seeing it through, because it is frankly *far more tolerable* than the lows that you are already experiencing… and which **further indulging the addiction** will continue to subject you to. This is because a). you'll know what to expect and b). you'll be in control and moving towards a wonderful vision of your life/yourself (living without limerence). Even if you do cry into your pillow for a few consecutive days, mourning this life chapter as you wave goodbye to accepting this LO's spell over you, the significance and purposefulness behind this emotional experience will render it oddly healing.

4. Only Radically Altering Your Subconscious Mind = Permanent Change

However, do not forget that stoicism and the active repression of your limerent feelings only work to attenuate current states of delusionality. While this line of action may be enough to snap you out of one particular limerent episode, it is ineffective at changing the configuration of your subconscious mind and thereby <u>will not prevent</u> future limerent episodes (that may well be worse). Even if you successfully employ 'no contact' and do forget about this LO, you will still radiate the same energy that screams "I need recognition and my needs met at all costs", which will invariably align you with similarly unhealthy romantic attachments (and, potentially, toxic people) over and over again. All future characters who exude intense spontaneity, authenticity, dominance, brusqueness or *whatever it is* that specifically meets the unmet needs that you harbour will seem like the last bottle of ice-cold Coca-Cola in the desert.

The very fact that you are **slipping into states of limerence** (and addicted to the wildness of the experience) reveals that you are carrying around significant psychological burdens that need to be treated. If you did not present with unmet needs and poorly integrated emotional wounds, you would not be interested in rogue LOs who orbit you but never show consistent interest, nor would you radiate the frequency that *they* are looking for. Even if your LO is not at all malicious, but is, rather, just someone who you feel you have 'connected with' in a specific way (whether a close friend or an acquaintance who just 'sparkles' to you uniquely), they are still providing you with <u>no real romantic connection</u>. The fact that <u>you nonetheless feel trapped in this situation</u> (and addicted to them) is, thus, reflective of you being **desperate to feel a certain way** regardless of *how much it costs you*. Desperate to have this person's energy in your life (even if only in the form of a weekly text message), because something very specific about them makes you, with your current unmet needs, feel 'good'.

The purpose of this book is to impart to you all the knowledge and tactics that you will need to completely eradicate the psychological underpinnings of limerence… from their roots. This will bestow upon you the ability to never cry over unrequited love again, to date exciting people (if you so wish) without having your emotions *controlled* by them, and to learn to tame and direct the **unruly ember of passion** that glows within you towards things and people that are actually worth your time.

5. Your Friends Won't Relate to Limerence

As you will have come to realise, not everyone experiences romance like you do and falls into limerence. In fact, a very small proportion of the population is genetically capable of the magical ideation and constant intrusive thoughts that the state entails, let alone the soaring highs and lows. As you progress deeper into the rawest phase of a limerent episode, a revelation of **the sheer rareness** of this state will creep up on you and may heighten your feelings of helplessness and resentment.

After all, your friends, even the unconventional, Bohemian and polyamorous ones, transition in and out of requited romantic bonds that seem to fill them with joy and serenity. It does not matter what those relationships look like, nor whether they even work out in the end, because you realise that that is not the point – the point is that they are in full control of their experience of romance in this reality. That it doesn't trigger horrendous emotional reactivity in them and consequently threaten their sanity.

While limerence has you physically nauseated, shaky, insomniac and prone to wailing into your pillow, they seem to only equate heartbreak with a few weeks of glumness and comfort-eating before surfacing, bright-eyed and unjaded, ready to take on the world again. It goes without saying that they never base the significance of their day on whether or not someone has sent them a message, nor do they ideate suicide over the allure of someone that they have never even been with. What could be so different about you that renders you prone to falling into unrequited love cycles that not only floor you emotionally, but also seem to plunge your body into a state of *systemic sickness*?

6. The Neurobiological Blueprint of Limerence

As with all mental illnesses, tendencies and personality traits, limerence is underpinned by a clear biological basis. We will not delve too deeply into the science behind neurotransmission in this book, but you must be aware of the following; the entire array of feelings that romance can induce in you can be traced back to the activity of neurons in certain brain regions. These neurons form microcircuits, where they orchestrate **complex patterns of activity** and send outputs to other areas of your brain to consolidate information and modulate your feelings, thoughts and, ultimately, behaviour.

The basis of this signalling is neurotransmission, involving chemical compounds being released by certain neurons onto other, nearby neurons at points of communication called synapses. The nature, strength and functionality of this neurotransmission depends on many different protein components and varies markedly depending on your genetics. The principal neurotransmitter systems that underpin limerence are the glutamatergic system, the

GABAergic system, the dopaminergic system, the noradrenergic system, the serotonergic system and the oxytocinergic system.

Your genome, which is the sum of all of the genetic information that you possess, includes all of the gene alleles that you have inherited from your parents. Many genes encode proteins that have nothing to do with limerence or mental health; for example, the KRT1 gene provides instructions for the production of keratin 1, a protein that forms part of human hair. A small proportion, however, encode the numerous **enzymes and receptor subcomponents** (which are all proteins) that make up the functional apparatus of each neurotransmitter system. The degree to which your brain possesses the 'equipment' to mediate smooth, seamless, well-regulated neurotransmitter production, signalling and metabolism will dictate how prone you are to obsession, mania, depression, and any other conceivable neurological phenomenon. Is it not beautiful and bizarre that we can trace every human emotion back to elements as small and impartial as proteins, even those that feel as momentous and spiritual as limerence?

7. Neural Communication In Action

To illustrate how neurons underprop emotional experiences, let's consider the functionality of the prefrontal cortex (PFC), which is involved in the consolidation of rich **episodic memories** involving your LO. When you picture them and feel a familiar limerent lurch in your stomach, or remember how the orange you ate before you last saw them tasted tart and floral, this is because your PFC has successfully consolidated your memories of them 'in context'. Such a memory faculty lets us complex beings collect autobiographical records beyond mere factual lists of what we have done, involving temporal information (i.e. when did this event/conversation take place) and a sense of self (i.e. you, an embodied individual, lived this experience). Unfortunately, it also allows your brain to throw intrusive memories your way, relentlessly reminding you just how glorious, nerve-wracking and heart-breaking your encounters with your LO have been.

Within a brain region like the PFC, the majority of the neurons are excitatory (referred to as projection neurons); these neurons project to *other* brain regions and release glutamate, the primary excitatory neurotransmitter, to regulate *their* activity. If they were uncontrolled, glutamatergic neurons would fire constantly and you would experience some of the effects of uncontrolled, run-away excitotoxicity: irrationality, seizures and cognitive damage. Fortunately, this is where the other major subpopulation of neurons comes in, known as inhibitory GABAergic interneurons. Their role is to control and **put a gate on excessive excitatory signalling**, GABA being the main inhibitory neurotransmitter in the brain. This GABA that they produce is released into spaces where it can bind to and stimulate projection neurons, making them probabilistically less likely to fire an action potential.

At this point, you'll be assimilating the idea that the excitation vs inhibition balance in your brain is a). very important in mental health, b). dependent upon which relevant neurotransmission-related proteins *your cells* can produce (including enzymes for neurotransmitter synthesis and metabolism and receptors for binding) and, hence, c). reflective of **the particular gene variants** you possess in your genome.

You may be wondering, however, where the neurotransmitters that you have always associated with 'love' come into this dynamic, computational representation of the brain.

8. Love Is A Neurochemical Concoction

We often talk about **dopamine, serotonin and noradrenaline** in the context of limerence; in contrast with glutamate and GABA, these are neuromodulators. The overwhelming majority of neurons produce the former two, with neuromodulators being produced by smaller nuclei (groups) of neurons in precise locations in the brain. Often acting diffusely across a whole-brain region, these neuromodulators bind to slow-acting receptors called 'G-protein coupled receptors' and, in doing so, affect the **conductivity of neurons** (their ability to fire action potentials and stimulate other neurons in their sphere of influence).

While the neurotransmitters glutamate and GABA are, respectively, strongly depolarising or hyperpolarising to the neuron (i.e. making it more or less likely to fire an action potential), neuromodulators like dopamine do not alter the neuron's membrane potential so significantly. Rather, they have a more subtle, clearly modulatory effect, only potentiating or attenuating responses evoked by our two principal neurotransmitters. In this way, they confer neural circuits with specificity and flexibility. Neuromodulators have evolved to allow neurons to fire at different rates and in different patterns in response to a vast range of similar, but distinct, stimuli. They allow us to feel an incredibly wide **range of sensations and states**, and to thrive as complex beings. After all, we humans need to be able to selectively focus and engage with tasks depending on how important we perceive them to be. This requires that we make rapid, prudent judgments and rapidly switch our focus. Being able to feel things with sharp acuity is a prerequisite to this type of adaptability, and it requires neuromodulation.

Different neurotransmitters elicit very different effects in neurons. As we have looked at, glutamate and GABA exert diametrically opposed effects on neuronal activity; the former is highly excitatory, and the latter highly inhibitory. The same can be said for different neuromodulators. Interestingly, however, a **single neuromodulator** will often impact *different neurons* differently, depending on which receptors that neuron expresses. Dopamine is a prime example, exciting neurons that contain the D1 dopamine receptor on their cell surface, and inhibiting ones that instead express the D2 dopamine receptor. It is also important to remember that, although the **functions of different brain regions** overlap far more than has traditionally been assumed, they do, nonetheless, differ. Naturally, therefore, the impact that neuromodulators have on your thoughts, feelings and behaviour can vary wildly depending on a). *where in the brain* they act, and on b). *which particular receptors* they act on within that region.

By acting at various different neural regions (and also, themselves, eliciting different effects in neurons), the various neuromodulators contribute to different components of the **emotional symptomatology of limerence**. The interplay of dopamine, serotonin, noradrenaline, oxytocin and vasopressin in various key brain regions (some of which we will take a look at) results in a bewildering, overwhelming emergent phenomenon: person addiction in its most intense form. As to avoid too many scientific chapters in a book designed to let you take action today, we will summarise the actions of the system most relevant to this state; keep reading to learn how **dopamine** signalling plays a pivotal role in sustaining and strengthening limerence, but *not* in the way that you may currently believe!

9. The Mesolimbic Dopaminergic Pathway

Produced by different neuronal nuclei in different regions of the midbrain, dopamine is inextricably linked to what we refer to as **hedonic gain**. This term describes our ability to enjoy an experience, get a 'hit' from it and be motivated on a visceral level to repeat it; all limerents with an interest in neuroscience will be able to deduce that this neuromodulator occupies a place of prominence in the pathophysiology of limerence, as the state involves the overwhelming desire to stay engaged with your LO and seek their attention, with withdrawal and dysphoria kicking in when you establish distance.

There are **four principal dopaminergic pathways**, mediating domains ranging from motor function to the coordination of executive control by the PFC. Here are the two that are relevant to limerence and addiction (NB: 'meso' refers to the fact that they originate in the midbrain, also known as the mesencephalon):

- The mesolimbic pathway: ventral tegmental area → nucleus accumbens and olfactory tubercle

- The mesocortical pathway: ventral tegmental area → prefrontal cortex

Stemming from the ventral tegmental area (VTA) and terminating in the **ventral striatum** of the forebrain basal ganglia (the nucleus accumbens and the olfactory tubercle), the mesolimbic dopaminergic pathway carries out the most important role in the generation of the reward-oriented cognition central to limerence. In other words, when dopamine is released by these VTA neurons and reaches the nucleus accumbens, this equates a 'reward' and strengthens the signalling of the neurons involved in the pathway. Activity in the nucleus accumbens is very closely correlated with the feeling of 'being in love', and, in limerence, with the ecstasy that you experience when you know that a meet-up (or phone call) with your LO is imminent.

Relating to what we have covered on genetics and neuron signalling, your ability to be limerent reflects **enhanced dopaminergic signalling** in this particular pathway. Yes, this separates you from a lot of people you know; your calm, level-headed flatmate who has the luxury of being able to mock the twin flame theory and boast that good food is more reinforcing to him than human attention will be *less prone* to **strong reward circuit activation** than you upon experiencing 'love'. However, a marked duality can be found in being more prone to latch onto people, so do not despair; it renders you more motivated by success and incentivised by goal-oriented pursuits than the average person. In later chapters, we will address how to tap into the magic behind your limerent disposition, permanently protect yourself from person addiction and pour this energy into other pursuits.

So far, we have not mentioned the second dopaminergic pathway that is implicated in limerence: the mesocortical pathway is closely associated with the mesolimbic pathway, despite having slightly different, nuanced roles relating to the management of reward value and the probability of the reward being delivered. While we are on the topic of neuroscience-related caveats, we ought to dispel a false notion: despite the pervasive ideas promoted by society and popular science articles, dopamine signalling in these two pathways is not *synonymous* with the buzz of a reward or the feelings of 'yumminess' and bliss. Remember, the brain is like a computer and not a slot machine; such clean-cut, causal associations between a). neural activity and b). behaviour are very rarely found. Let us proceed!

10. Time to Leave Behind The 'Dopamine = Pleasure' Moniker

In the late 1990s, leading neuroscientists confirmed that the theory that 'pleasure experienced is directly proportional to the amount of dopamine swimming around in the reward pathways' was overly-simplified and incorrect. They did well, for in contrast with the popular pseudoscientific axiom that claims that 'all you need to do to feel good is to boost your dopamine with X superfoods', dopamine alone is *not* responsible for the ability to enjoy something and catch a 'buzz'. For that reason, I recommend supplements like NAC that aid the modulation of various neurotransmitter systems and heal brain inflammation rather than mega-dosing any one compound.

Dopamine is very much *relevant* to the **experience of bliss**, indeed, and untreated Parkinson's sufferers are often depressed and apathetic. But, is this neuromodulator capable of explaining the entire experience of something feeling 'rewarding'? No. If individuals are allowed to choose between sucrose water and distilled water after global dopamine depletion (i.e. leaving them with no neural dopamine), they will still opt for the former and find it more pleasurable to consume. This alone shows that the the experience of a dreamy 'reward' that taps into our senses cannot be *solely mapped to* the impulses of neurons in our two key dopaminergic pathways.

The more evidence, the better, so I am going to summarise some more results for you (all the references can be found at the back of this book). In concordance with the sucrose study results, a study involving amphetamine users ascertained that mesolimbic pathway activity correlated more closely with the user ***desiring* the drug** than with the surging euphoria experienced actually upon ingesting it. Furthermore, certain populations of dopaminergic neurons in the midbrain are activated when an experience is aversive; this form of dopaminergic activity is, by definition, inversely correlated with bliss!

We now believe that, instead of generating euphoric experiences in itself, dopamine release is crucial for the formation of pathways that represent the **'salience', i.e. noteworthiness**, of a stimulus. It trains the brain to seek a particular reward depending on its predicted value, and this representational coding, in turn, allows us to become firmly addicted. Of course, activity in the two major reward-related dopaminergic pathway *does* correlate with the obtainment of all rewards, whether they be chocolate, romantic reciprocation or video-game points. You can observe this easily using fMRI imaging; people in love and people experiencing other rewards possess high metabolic activity in the VTA, nucleus accumbens and PFC. But, dopamine's role is best conceptualised as being *computational*; it really encodes a signal that allows you to learn that the reward exists and is worth your effort, hence establishing 'reward-seeking behaviour'.

Thus, since we now understand this caveat regarding the traditional dopamine = reward dogma, I do not want any of you to grow fearful imagining all the 'excess dopamine' that must be floating around your brain whenever you experience a limerent upswing. It is almost certain that very strong signalling will have occurred in the pathways mentioned to project you to these heights of addiction, but not in the sense that every microscopic drop of dopamine is matched by a relatively-potent burst of adrenaline and joy. How artificial, odd and downright undesirable the notion of reward could get if we conceptualised it in this overly simplified way!

The goal of this neurobiological section is to provide you with an analytical and edifying take on the emotions that have dominated your life for a significant period of time. This does not mean that I want you to *worry about* the **neurochemical basis of this condition** or to excessively self-medicate, for this is unnecessary and would be barking up the wrong tree. As will be clear when we tackle how to alter your self-concept and truly become limerence-immune (despite your genetic propensity to the state), the most powerful recovery tools are not those that try and balance the activity individual neurotransmitter systems. They are those that alter your thoughts, beliefs and your self-concept; in response to these incredibly effective psychological interventions and associated behaviour changes, **the brain heals, modulates and optimises** its neuronal activity/neurotransmission *all by itself.*

Trying to alter the way that your brain regions communicate to permanently cure limerence would be like looking in the mirror and trying to take a photo of yourself smiling without prior movement of your face muscles. You may be able to grab your cheeks and hold an artificial smile for a little while, but soon enough, the root cause (those lazy facial muscles) will result in you once again looking serious. Neuroscientific understanding of human emotional afflictions is powerful, enlightening and necessary, but real human *improvement* lies in controlling what we can control: the suggestible, receptive chamber that is **the subconscious mind**.

Once you learn to do this, freedom will be yours – everything will sort itself out to allow you to step into a healthy version of yourself: the emotional eating, anxiety-induced undereating, overactive reward system activation and insufficient PFC control over the 'limbic', emotional brain will all be normalised for you.

11. Dopamine is More About Anticipation Than Reward

So, we now know that dopaminergic activity is closely correlated with that limerent 'rush', but it is not the only factor responsible for those wonderful, mystical feelings that you feel when your LO looks your way. The role of this modulator gets even more nuanced when we look at well-established addictions, because we see that dopaminergic activity (in the mesolimbic and mesocortical pathways, of course) does not just occur *when the reward is obtained.* In fact, once **the reward contingencies** of this particular stimulus are known, i.e. in what scenarios 'gains', 'losses' or 'mixed outcomes' are likely, dopamine is predominately released during <u>anticipation</u>.

This will make sense to you on an intuitive level; a child contently enjoys a chocolate sundae from the local Italian café and the resulting sugar high, but when does she truly jump with joy? When her dad *announces* that he is taking her for the treat, and on the way to the van, clutching his hand while she skips. Similarly, despite conversations and exchanges with your LO initially hitting you hard and feeling too good to be true, consider this – once you are deep in the pits of limerence, what is it that *actually* guarantees you the best feeling? What soothes your malaise, sets you up for the day and makes you feel strong again, after days of no contact and crying spells?

Once you are weeks/months into a tough limerent episode that has you in its jaws, you will experience the most marked high <u>when you believe that you *will* secure time</u> with your LO. I (lamentably, for limerents are always engrossing people!) do not know your name, your age or the gender that you identify with, but I do know that your brain is controlled on a primitive level by dopamine circuits that mediate interesting evolutionary roles regarding reward. It just so happens that evolution has conferred to us the ability to gain more pleasure from knowing a reward *is coming* than from actually experiencing it.

Imagine that your LO is a colleague, and you suddenly hear that they will be sat next to you at the Christmas party. **Your mood skyrockets**; you feel productive, full of purpose and blessed during the day, and crack jokes with people you're not normally even that keen on. On the way home, you dawdle around some shops to decide which gorgeous outfit you are going to splash out on for this momentous occasion – the world is once again your oyster, and you see colour in everything.

Of course, actually sitting next to your LO and talking to them at the party will be great (if they are on friendly terms with you, and this bond is not entirely fantasy-based), but that high will be *nothing* compared to what you experience the moments following your discovery that you are 'guaranteed access' to them soon. The anticipation and assurance that you *will* see this person, that they *will* talk to you soon and bathe you in their sacred, golden attention, is precisely what slingshots you towards those **alarming heights of limerent euphoria** that make this pathology so difficult to escape. Once a person addiction is established, the gratification that the reward *itself* offers is mood-stabilising and pleasant, but it is the afterthought compared to the rush that you experience during the build-up (unless, of course, you do not receive this reward at all in the end. In that case, you certainly will know about it and will be flooded with despair, grief and a sense of impending doom).

At this point, I know that some of you will be unconvinced by the depiction of the actual 'reward' of your LO's attention being less enjoyable than your anticipation of it. You may have some scenes in mind that felt like pure, rare magic; maybe you and your LO shared a drunk, philosophical conversation and both confessed that you'd love to move to Russia one day, or perhaps a Facebook exchange about your shared hatred of a mutual acquaintance left you swimming through treacly bliss for hours. Not to forget, some people do *actually date* their LOs before the love turns unrequited – it might be that you and your LO dined in restaurants together, discussed your dreams of raising a feline family together and kissed for hours while passers-by flicked envious eyes your way.

If you *have* experienced sublime things with your LO in real life, your internal voice will be raising the following, very valid point of interjection: does *anticipation alone* really grant us stronger highs than actual time spent with our LOs? How can this be true when some limerents struggle most with their inability to let go of real, precious memories that they have excessively romanticised?

Think about it: what do the above examples of 'real interactions' with a LO have in common that makes them so euphoria-begetting? They all produce the illusion that **you and your LO have a *future* together**, and that you are not going to 'lose access' to them. Yes, a date with your LO involving long conversations is *only so magical* because your brain is sighing a sigh of relief and thinking "this person is mine; I am secured a long future of my needs being met. Of them making me feel great." By nature, all <u>limerent bliss</u> is **synonymous with you anticipating future times** with your LO, i.e. future rewards. Limerence is really all about finding someone who uniquely complements your psychological issues, enjoying the overpowering euphoria that occurs when you start to connect, and then spending months or years doing all that you can to *ensure your permanent access* to them (in vain and to your utter detriment).

So that you fully grasp the implications of all of this, I want you to imagine the following: how would you feel if you were eating dinner with your LO and they told you that they were moving to a different company/country/would somehow never see you again? Regardless of how well you two were connecting in that moment, you'd be automatically jolted out of your elevated state and sent into a dismal frame of mind. You'd be depressed, potentially even tearful – and certainly bombarded by mental imagery of you having to bleakly and painfully pull yourself through the next few months.

However, if your LO then added that they 'might actually **just spend ten months** abroad/elsewhere, and *then return*' because they 'could probably never truly say goodbye' to the city and the people in their life, your spirits would soar again. And, then crash when you realised that they might not *actually come back* in ten months' time... that people are often capricious, and their plans flexible. What if your LO doesn't come back – if you never see them again? But, they've told you they probably will, and they've proven themself to be fairly true to their word in the past, haven't they – and they **do love this city**, don't they?

But, then again, they're likely to meet splendid people wherever they go, and are more than capable of building a new life elsewhere and never turning back. At the end of the day, you *know* that your permanent access to their energy **isn't guaranteed**.

Oh, how agonising it is to be limerent... how delusional it makes you, clutching at the possibility of future enmeshment with your LO while convincing yourself that you two share a functional connection.

However, viewing it like this (involving you *craving* them and calculating how you can influence them to always be there for you and never want anything/anyone else) is a very, very potent way to **snap yourself out of the soulmate delusion** – out of the idea that this connection is, for you, the most 'beautiful, perfect, natural' expression of romance. No one that you feel this way towards is ever going to align with you in a meaningful way, nor should they – unfortunately, this is not how any type of relationship works. In this state, you're as far away from a **playful, abundant mentality** as you could possibly be, and you're doing yourself a massive injustice – you're fixating on a target that cannot be moved, and are wasting your mental, emotional and spiritual energy. You cannot move the needle here, because people cannot be controlled in the way that you currently wish you could control your LO. So, it's utterly imperative that you commit to overcoming this. That you instead chase *your own* success, bliss, and freedom.

After all, imagine if **one of your friends** tried to secure your time, attention and energy in this way. If one of your siblings, or even your own parents, did. Imagine if you felt that *anyone* in your life was hyper-focused on *where you'd be* in the future... and that you induced crazy, turbulent emotions in them – emotions that made them dream about throwing away their entire life to follow you wherever you went. Imagine if you sensed that they wanted to freeze time whenever you two were together, regardless of how you treated them. Imagine them desiring to keep you exactly as you were in the moment... giving them **a limitless supply** of your interest, admiration and attention.

Because limerence isn't just about wanting to lock this person down in a particular geographical location, that much we all know. Continuing with our previous, suitably lamentable example, imagine that **your LO did come back** ten months later after all, *but with a new significant other* they'd met abroad. Would you be jumping for joy, as you anticipated you would be? Most definitely not. Nor would you be if they were single and free but somehow *less engaged with you...* disinterested in the deep conversations you two had before, and a little colder. You'd be absolutely heartbroken (and potentially resentful), receiving none of the 'pick me up' that you so deeply craved.

You see, limerence is a dark entity – you're needy while limerent, but also highly manipulative. This isn't your fault in the slightest, of course; it's a loathsome condition that 'corners' you into **acting entirely incongruently** with your nature, trying to force someone to be there physically, mentally and emotionally in a particular, unique way that *makes you feel good*. It distances you from your own intrinsic sense of value, putting you in 'seller' mode – you constantly wonder what you can show/'sell' your LO to keep them where they are, as they are, and interested in you. Life must involve you assessing people in 'buyer' mode, too – you want to switch between the two modes in equal parts, also wondering whether people are a good fit for *you*. Qualifying people, and letting them qualify you. Limerence is, by definition, a scarcity mentality, so it distances you from so many things that make you the person that you are: your discrepancy, your natural desire to judge what's right for you/not commit to things too quickly, your self-respect…it makes you think *"what can I give/do/become/sell, so I don't lose my LO?"*

But worry not, for you are in no way bound to this state. Limerence is entirely curable – when you become a version of yourself that your LO (or any future LO) *can't* make feel so problematically euphoric and addicted, none of this madness can occur. It simply evaporates from your reality. Free from the artificial highs, the lows will no longer be triggered, and you'll become incapable of displaying ingratiating, humiliating behaviour towards anyone. You'll be once again confident, relaxed and living in the moment, with an incredibly resilient sense of self and a lust for life itself.

Later on in this book, you'll learn exactly how to accomplish this transformation. For the time being, however, we are going to keep exploring the biological basis of limerence, just to provide you with the satisfaction of *knowing what it is* in tangible, scientific terms.

12. Evolutionary Explanation: Why Does Anticipation of A Reward Win?

Now, back to dopamine and how it primarily provides you with a rush in anticipation of seeing your LO. I hope your mind is as blown by the insight broken down in the previous chapter as mine was when I first elucidated it. To add even more reputability to this already-scientifically-backed concept of 'the *anticipation* of a reward feeling better than actually experiencing it', imagine what would happen if this were *not* the case. If we all basked in joy and felt amazing whenever we experienced any positive stimuli, in addition to wreaking havoc on our nervous systems (you will learn why we must habituate to rewards in Chapter 18), this would not be conducive to survival.

Imagine a hungry chimpanzee securing a banana; if she experienced the strongest, longest-lasting joy and motivation *upon eating it*, she would a). probably consequentially dance around and waste the calories consumed and b). would grow complacent and would be far less likely than other chimpanzees to seek out more bananas. The same applies to romance. In such a dynamic world, where members of all mammalian species occupy multiple roles (e.g. self-preservation, guarding the nest, caring for pups and/or baby humans), pursuing a mate requires individuals to take some degree of action. If the odd conversation with your special someone generated **more euphoria in you** than an exciting message that revealed their deep interest in you (and which revealed that *future escalations* in the connection were imminent), you would not be bothered to see through the progression of the relationship.

In other words, if you were not wired for 'reward anticipation' to hit you as hard as it does, you would not be motivated to act in a way that allowed *any romantic connections* to unfold. If the human brain were not orchestrated in this way, regardless of how much joy was inspired in you upon seeing your partner, there would be no way to incentivise you to seek future access to this same person. Nor would you be driven to buy food, to speak to anyone you like platonically *or* romantically, to take care of your appearance or to delay any form of gratification.

If you were constantly, viscerally overwhelmed by joy and ecstasy upon sitting on your sofa and contemplating your small flat, you would never forgo an afternoon of sunbathing to attend house viewings. The anticipation of enjoying a new home and the upgrades in aesthetics, social status and comfort would not more thrilling than what you currently experience. If you came across a fun, intelligent new person, even if you saw great platonic potential, you would never be moved enough by the prospect of a real friendship to text them and invite them over. As a consequence, you would have zero friends and would not benefit from the emotional wellbeing and physical protection that an intimate platonic circle rewards you with. This would render you very vulnerable if you were a **primitive human living off the grid**, rather than in a safe town or city.

This fascinating neuroscientific axiom is neatly encapsulated by the following statement: the brain does not want you to feel good or the time, *nor can it* orchestrate a perpetual state of bliss – it wants to motivate you to keep yourself alive, healthy and in a position to reproduce.

Naturally, this is a result of natural selection, for reasons that the aforementioned examples illustrate nicely. We would not be functional, let alone thrive, if we were not wired to feel the best 'hits' during the *mere anticipation* of a great reward. There is no escaping this, nor the fact that euphoria cannot be our baseline state. We *all* have to deal with some duller, quieter, sadder moments. People who take drugs to feel better and 'raise their baseline state', however, try and circumvent this reality. Whilst transiently working, this ironically and tragically results in them experiencing a). far more marked peaks and troughs and b). a more intense version of the aforementioned phenomenon: 'you get to feel good/okay when you find your reward, but I will only let you feel ***amazing*** when you know that more is coming'.

You only need to watch a documentary on heroin or crystal meth users to see how substance abuse curates an exaggerated and destructive caricature of dopamine's natural, survival-promoting effects. Of course, limerence can be conceptualised as a similar state of full-blown addiction, involving desperate attempts to guarantee yourself 'more' of your LO.

13. We Are Cerebral Beings, But Still Animals; Let That Comfort You

As has already been mentioned, the primary purpose of this neurobiological section is to allow you to view limerence more objectively. Knowing that we can identify the activity of various neurotransmitters that coincide with limerent feelings that seem so **ethereal and spiritual** reduces limerence to what it is: a complex pathology. Furthermore, exploring the computational role of dopamine in full allows you to temporarily transcend your mental state and project yourself towards the recovery trajectory. This is because learning that you are specifically-programmed to feel thrilled when you think that future bonding experiences with your LO are coming (i.e. upon anticipation) translates limerence into visceral, primitive terms – it breaks the spell.

At the end of the day, while labelling limerence a 'psychic affliction', 'heartbreak' or a 'spiritual dilemma' is not inaccurate *per se* (for those are just different lenses through which we can attempt to understand the world), initially educating yourself on its neurobiological correlates offers unparalleled healing benefits.

After all, I do not want you to suppress or deny anything, but I do want you to identify your emotions with precision and deem them something limiting and problematic, rather than indulging in them and their mysteriousness. You need to comprehend limerence from various angles to fully recover, hence why I am weaving aspects of all implicated fields into this book, but **a unique power** lies in understanding just how **primitive and biologically explicable** this addiction is. Limerence is engaging basic, limbic neural machinery within you that would promote your survival if we were navigating the wild. Our ancestors who were able to apply the same neuroticism and unwavering focus to fruit-foraging, hunting or to rounding up their various children survived; for this reason, limerence-producing genes stay with us today, despite them wreaking havoc on us. Fortunately, they gift us with special intellectual faculties and idiosyncratic ways of progressing through life, too (see Chapter 32).

14. The Oxytocin-Vasopressin Pathway: Pair-Bonding and Tenderness

Oxytocin and vasopressin are the peptide molecules responsible for the feelings of intimacy and attachment that grow when we are in love, regardless of whether we are transitioning into a real relationship or **merely fantasising** about a LO who does not feel the same way for us. On its own, the oxytocin pathway is responsible for non-specific social attention and reward, while the vasopressin pathway pertains to social avoidance, aggression and anxiety. These two molecules evolved from a shared genetic source, and their addition to mammalian genomes reflects the growing complexity of all species over time and the increased need for social specificity. For example, pair-bonding, maternal aggression, social receptibility and the desire to defend our family and friends are all contingent on the ability to not only distinguish between 'them and us' (i.e. who we consider part of our group and who we do not) but to also **adhere to the rules** generated by an ever-changing society. For example, if human monogamy suddenly became societally shunned and punishable, perhaps the result would be a shift in the gene pool and, eventually, more polyamorous individuals.

At least for the time being (!), partnering-up is far from unnatural for most people. Evolutionary processes that have conferred to us, as humans, the ability to interact with, 'latch onto' and experience partners in nuanced and complex ways have given rise to a distinct, integrated system involving both peptides. Allowing us to engage in sexual practices *selectively*, and to bond with *specific* partners that take our fancy, the oxytocin-vasopressin pathway is highly active when limerence has us in its grips.

This is particularly reflected in the fact that fully-developed limerence feels like true love, and *is* a form of love, albeit unwise, fruitless and ill-directed love. While the experience is predominantly electric, thrilling and cut by a dreaded sensation of urgency, leaving you prepared to lie about your talents or become someone else if it may give you a chance to be with your LO (operation 'grab this special person!'), many limerents do end up transitioning towards wanting to display their feelings in *tender, unselfish* romantic ways too. If you find yourself occasionally thinking that 'all you want is to stroke your LO's hair and comfort them', realise that this is a fib (as you will always want more attention, more contact and more 'hits'), albeit a convincing one, orchestrated by the oxytocin-vasopressin pathway.

Receptors for these two peptides are abundant in areas of the brain involved in complex social functions. Among these are the **nucleus accumbens** (the terminal point of the mesolimbic pathway, a.k.a. the brain region implicated in addiction that we discussed in Chapter 9), the **cortex** and the **amygdala**. Aside from occupying a key role in the generation of learned fear, the amygdala (plural - you possess one in both of your brain hemispheres) is an almond-shaped brain region found deep within the medial temporal lobe. It is implicated in not only aggression and fear, but also in love, particularly **unstable love** that involves intermittent reward and strong emotionality. These peptide receptors are also found in the nucleus accumbens (due to its implication in reward and reinforcement).

Can all sentimental impulses always be traced exclusively back to activity in this pathway? No; as always, we are breaking down very complex neurobiological phenomena that, due to their importance to reproduction and the survival of our species, evolution has prioritised and optimised over hundreds of thousands of years. No single neuromodulator, pathway or brain region can explain, in entirety, your deep, primitive urges to emulate your LO and spend time with them, nor your grief over not being the first person that they run to when their elderly dog passes away.

In our chapters on enigmatic dopamine, I touched on the fact that dopamine alone can reinforce addictive behaviours, but *cannot wholly explain* the urge you feel to be with your LO or the 'highs' that they provide you with. Similarly, the oxytocin-vasopressin pathway is important in generating feelings of intimacy in limerence, whether real or entirely illusory. It does this in response to input from either *real or imagined* **bonding** with your LO being processed by the brain. However, just as dopamine is far from being the only player in the neurochemical cascade that results in you feeling 'hooked' to your LO, feeling 'intimately bonded' to your LO requires more than *just* input from oxytocin and vasopressin.

Consider this right now; can you genuinely harbour warm, tender feelings without wanting to do something about them (even if it be something as innocent as sending your LO 'happy birthday'), or without experiencing some visceral sensations? We may claim we can, but even when we believe that we 'unconditionally love' a LO and have 'set them free', we are lit **up by the idea** of phoning them, or even by seeing that they have been promoted via a Facebook post. Such cognitive processes require far more than just oxytocin and vasopressin, relying on the combined effects of dopamine and many other signallers.

All limerent symptoms, revelations and feelings, whether indignant or exuberant, are the product of the interplay between many different types of signalling in different brain areas, mediated by a rich array of distinct signalling molecules. What can be said, however, is that some key, well-understood pathways will be far more implicated in some facets of limerence than others, hence why there *is* value in stripping limerence down and studying these individually as we have done. Appreciating the **neuroscientific basis of your obsessive romantic feelings** (and the fact that they are the result of hundreds of thousands of years of evolution) leaves you better equipped to see past the delusionality that the state attempts to forcibly feed you with.

15. Why Do We Label Limerence? Can Love Really Be Pathological?

When I started this book, I knew I was committing to exhaustively analysing limerence from multiple different angles in order to entirely quench your thirst for knowledge and mental expansion. I'm aware that the burden of limerence will have you desperately seeking information, recovery strategies and spiritual support, and to top it off, that your neural makeup makes you a naturally curious and discerning individual. Consistent with your nature, you will want to consider all the philosophical dilemmas that limerence raises *before* committing to leaving it behind.

One of these major philosophical dilemmas is whether we should analyse limerence so methodically or even attempt to treat it, when it bathes us in emotions that feels so significant and spiritual. After all, love (and the lucid mania it can charge us with) is one of the most potent sources of inspiration, catalysing poetry, music, travel escapades and self-transformation all over the world. When we only have a certain number of decades on this planet, why try to actively avoid love-induced sickness if it feels so important and sentimental?

As I have covered in Chapter 2, these concerns are completely valid but can be dismissed as **a mere side-effect** of the very addiction that you are trapped in. Someone obese and addicted to sugar may be convinced that life would be miserable if they tamed their unbridled consumption of food, because they are currently trapped in the behavioural addiction of consuming, getting a reward, attempting to recover, feeling withdrawals and finally throwing in the towel and bingeing on cookies. It is only natural that they respond to promises that they will be able to go for four-hour long hikes with friends without fretting about their next snack with utter disbelief. This example may be a crude depiction of addiction entrapment, but you are currently experiencing the romantic equivalent of this, and are naturally equally unable to comprehend that a sparky, strong and motivated You is waiting for you on the other side of these highs and lows. Let the conclusion of Chapter 2 comfort and greatly excite you; you can leave behind the fear that recovery is going to plant you in an austere, excitement-void life that does not suit you, because there is simply no risk of this when we grow into superior versions of ourselves.

Jolting back to our existential quandary over whether limerence is truly bad, it's crucial that you realise that *all* of the various ways that we romanticise the **emotional upswings of pathological love** are equally *incapable of justifying* them. But, the mere fact that limerence is an addiction that <u>entails much more lows than highs</u> is potentially the most convincing reminder that it cannot be indulged – that it is a damaging behavioural pattern that must be escaped. Subjecting yourself to so much pain, and so unnecessarily, will never be admissible or fair to yourself.

After all, I take it for granted that you have had some grimy first-hand experience with the compromising, humiliating and demobilising agony that being emotionally-enmeshed with LOs submits to you. Therefore, I do not need to explain the downsides of living with these highs and lows. However, I do wish to draw your attention to just how *transient* (and meaningless, in the grand scheme of things) the euphoric upswings of limerence are, and how leaving it untreated condemns you to a life sentence of permanently aching for what you will never hold onto.

In order for me to be able to do this effectively, we will need to consider the progression of an individual limerent episode. The next four chapters will be dedicated to looking at how limerence unfolds, starting from the **initial glimmer**, and ending in agonising, entrenched **dependence** that feels (but luckily *never is*) impossible to escape.

16. The Initial Glimmer and The Urge to Be Engulfed

As with any other addiction involving an unpredictable reward system (i.e. your LOs behaviour towards you), limerence starts on a high note when you come across a LO and sense something in them that your brain equates with spiritual *inevitability*. "We're just meant to be together in some way, shape or form," you will think, even if not on a conscious level. They seem instantly and categorically wondrous to you, and you cannot comprehend why others who interact with them in your mutual circles aren't equally bewitched by their presence. While hindsight and wisdom allow you to elucidate *which of their traits* must have resonated with you and fed you what you craved at the time, when you come across this person and experience the 'limerent glimmer', such logical, detached intuition is impossible.

As the limerence bubble closes around you while you remain blissfully unaware, it won't dawn on you that their towering height and self-assured voice is making you feel safe and cherished, something you never felt as a child, or that their **interesting juxtaposition** of femininity and brash outspokenness provides you with the very dose of colour and chaos that your jaded soul needs. Instead, you will feel an enormous force vigorously expelling itself from you and urging you to do all that you can to enmesh with them entirely. You fall hook, line and sinker, unbothered that there may be no one there to catch you (or, perhaps more realistically, you are pushed off a cliff unaware that no one *can* catch you).

While I prefer to use a basis of neurobiology to help people objectify their suffering, limerence can be stripped down and summarised as 'the desire for enmeshment at the cost of anything'; the limerent's ultimate goal is *complete spiritual and emotional engulfment* by their LO. Of course, the root cause of this urge is this LO's unique ability to shield you from the unmet needs, unfulfillment, psychological damage, and negative beliefs that you carry around.

A good way to visualise this is that these psychological issues of yours form part of a poorly constructed Rubik's cube, leaving you with a difficult attachment style that does not apply well to adult life. It is only natural that the pieces that complement yours (i.e. what your LO provides you with on a psychological level) will be equally aberrant.

We will look at LOs, how they typically act, and what type of connections limerents typically fall into with them in Chapter 29. However, I want to remind you now that indulging in the fantasy bond that you have with your LO is self-sabotage to the maximum, because they are not *perfect* for you or 'the only one for you' – not **scientifically, emotionally or spiritually**. They simply have the specific nature that complements and *softens* the painful, deeply rooted psychological issues that you are walking around with. Facing up to this truth as early as possible in your recovery process is essential. It will quieten your limbic (emotional) brain's desires to cling onto the twin flame illusion, and help you realise that your life really would be better without limerence at its crux.

Let's get back to discussing the initial phase of limerence; evolutionarily designed to immerse you in a pool of velvety, syrupy delusion, it is what initially 'revs up' your most vulnerable emotions and gets the ball rolling. It is what locks you into limerence... into a tenacious, destructive addiction to another human being's attention and reciprocation, and longing for their undying love.

17. The Honeymoon Phase

Fleeting and sugary by nature, the honeymoon phase of a limerent episode does not last long, but will be eternally romanticised and sentimentalised by the limerent as long as they remain emotionally hooked onto that same individual. This first phase is typically when real communication or signs of potential reciprocation are occurring, and each of these 'hits' will send euphoria coursing through your veins in a way that is completely akin to the actions of a stimulant drug. Text messages or smiles from your LO will send you up to the clouds, and this dopaminergic high may also impulse you to look at yourself in the mirror more, buy yourself little gifts, get yourself into prime physical shape and immerse yourself in hobbies and content that your LO enjoys (or would admire).

After all, **an evolutionary switch** has been flicked in your brain; your desire not only to enmesh but also pair-bond romantically with your LO has grabbed control of the reins. And, as we have seen in the context of dopaminergic signalling, this is all about sweet, protective, titillating <u>anticipation</u>.

Primitive, pro-reproductive biochemical cascades make planning for a future with your LO in it not only motivate and uplift you, but also seem entirely rational, prudent and necessary. Oh, does the brain love a scarcity mindset and to make you feel that you will never find an intimate mental connection again, but this is all lies. The tendency to feel that food, mates and resources are *scarce and precious* is always going to be evolution's gold standard, and it is preserved in every animal that can be found on this planet.

However, in this modern reality paradigm we live in, we do not have to physically fight for food in the supermarket, nor do we have to partner up as soon as possible if we want children so as to avoid being killed by bears before we get a chance to reproduce. Therefore, **real magic and satisfaction** are garnered from realising that we are the creators of our destiny, and that life's better offerings are abundant. Plus, even if interesting people weren't plentiful, would it not be a huge mistake to waste years crying over one who intermittently rewards us and never offers us any consistent recognition?

18. The Crystallisation Phase

We all know that rewards become less exciting when they are given often; the habituation phenomena is a key mechanism of the nervous system, extending beyond just dopaminergic signalling. We habituate to any drug that we consistently receive, as the brain does not and cannot conduct the signalling that produces euphoria for prolonged periods in response to the **same, unchanged stimulus**. Neural homeostatic mechanisms work to ensure that networks of neurons maintain their activity around a desirable 'set point' – if such an adaptation did not occur, your brain would suffer from circuit instability, uncontrolled excitation and consequent issues like epilepsy and horrific anxiety.

An example of one of these adaptive mechanisms is an **individual neuron's** ability to increase or decrease the number of receptors that it expresses, making it more or less 'excitable' by neurotransmitters that are being released onto it. For example, let's consider someone who **drinks coffee every morning**. Their neurons will eventually make themselves less responsive to glutamate by reducing their number of postsynaptic ionotropic glutamate receptors; many other modifications of the same nature will also be triggered in other neurotransmitter systems. In turn, this person will *not be able to* permanently experience the same sharp, lucid productivity from coffee, unless they take a long enough 'tolerance break' to allow their neurons to undo these alterations and reach baseline again. This decreased reactivity to a drug such as caffeine can be visualised through fMRI; the more the same drug/stimulus is experienced, the less activity will be seen in certain brain regions that were initially activated very strongly.

Of course, as we first started to explore in Chapter 6, we are all extremely different physiologically and, therefore, psychologically; some of us are more prone to experiencing abnormal states like mania and psychosis (which represent poor regulation and flexibility of neural circuits) than others. In this sense, everything is relative – some people will experience potent initial euphoria from certain things that others will **never get a marked 'hit' from** or be able to become 'addicted to' (whether they be compounds, like caffeine, or experiences like love/thrill-seeking/gambling).

However, regardless of your personal genetics and neural makeup, your brain will have **its own 'set points'** like the ones we have outlined in this chapter. This means that any substance/experience that affects *you* intensely will start to affect you less and less, until (in the case of continued/chronic exposure) *you need it to feel 'normal'* (dependence). You know where this is going – this means that your limerence-prone brain will always alter its functional properties and signalling/output upon prolonged exposure to delicious limerent highs. The result will be that a). these highs don't feel quite as powerful as they used to, and b). you will start to feel low without them.

19. Dependence: What Felt Good Yesterday Is *Needed* Today (and Isn't Enough Tomorrow)

So, we have seen that dynamic neural adaptations constantly strive to maintain a state of homeostasis and maintain the brain's output as even as possible. In other words, once you are addicted to a substance or experience, your brain will not work in the same way without it (until the vice is successfully overcome). As with limerence, genetics play a huge role in drug metabolism; some people barely experience a pick-me-up buzz from caffeine, while others report that it feels like a strong stimulant to them. However, anyone who does respond to tea or coffee will soon find that their addiction becomes more about drinking it to feel okay and awake, rather than to feel great. This is an exemplar example of drug habituation turning into **dependence**, another incredibly important constituent of the limerent experience.

The neural basis of becoming 'dependent' on your LOs addiction, your sugary morning smoothie or the Redbull that you initially started drinking as a student is virtually identical to that of the habituation I have described. When the activity of your central nervous system is consistently perturbed due to a stimulus being presented over and over again, your brain's line of action is to *attenuate its impact*. Since doing so requires it to alter the physical makeup and functionality of the neurons involved, they will act in a suboptimal way when the stimulus is not available. Eventually, if the addiction is not nipped in the bud, you will feel miserable nearly all of the time that you do not see, speak to or fantasise about your LO, only intermittently feeling 'normal' and stable when you cave in and do one of these things.

I refer to this as the crystallisation phase of limerence, because it is person addiction in its grimmest, most destructive and fully developed form. If you are identifying with this description and realising your limerent episode entails a great degree of dependence, recovery is of the utmost importance. I realise how insurmountable and impossible it will seem, but you can leave this behind, just as a plucky, committed heroin addict can physiologically detox from the drug, commit to healing the psychological wounding that made the lulling high resonate with them strongly and give themself their best chance. We all deserve our best chance.

20. Psychological Factors Prime You For Limerence

Now that we have analysed the prominent neurobiological symptomatology of the limerent experience, I am going to delve into the psychological factors that result in someone who is genetically prone to limerence actually *falling into* limerence. We will be now looking at the emotions, weaknesses and desires involved in the state, leaving talk of neurotransmission (that naturally *does* underpin all of these processes) behind. Naturally, these psychological faculties are inextricably intertwined with spirituality; we humans are driven by our minds to make sense of the world, and we weave up narratives in an attempt to explain the ineffable and bizarre feelings that we are capable of. For this reason, you will see me touching on concepts such as the Law of Assumption and the creative power of the subconscious mind as we progress into this section.

To clarify, the multi-faceted analysis of a state like limerence is essential in terms of understanding and treating it. I had to explain the basis of 'being limerence-prone' to you in terms of genetics and neurotransmission, but if I were to be pushing the pure neurobiology viewpoint on you and ignoring psychology, I would be going down the line of recommending that you seek pharmaceuticals. Apart from eating a healthy, refined-sugar-free diet and taking some truly transformative supplements like NAC (as I write about on my website), I do not recommend attempting to **alter your brain chemistry**. Despite psychology being a 'softer; science than neuroscience, it is equally *if not more* important in the transition away from limerence and towards emotional freedom.

After all, not everyone who has the neurobiological makeup to experience obsessionality and euphoric highs becomes limerent. I want to stress that these psychological points of weakness that I am going to teach you how to abolish are, for someone of your nature, the difference between a). living a life dictated by unrequited love and person addiction and b). living a curious, adventurous, fulfilling life of which you are the conscious creator. Genetically-speaking, I possess the limerent mentality to the absolute maximum and visited hell and back in my teenage years and early-mid twenties, yet learnt to completely master my own subconscious mind and eliminate the psychological elements that were manifesting these appalling limerent episodes in my life. I am now incapable of ever falling for the erratic and inconsistent people I used to pedestal, and often prefer to be single because I find my own time so uniquely fulfilling. However, when I do wish to enter a romantic relationship that is aligned with my professional goals, there is no resistance and I effortlessly attract love that is stimulating but genuine.

The *main* two areas of relevance in your transformation here are:

- **Unmet needs**
- **Detrimental belief systems**

When a limerent-prone individual, young or old, is dealing with some issues that fall into any of these two categories, they will, without exception, attract LOs who shimmer to them like liquid gold. Wondering why these limerent episodes are 'happening to them', or why they 'attract LOs with personality disorders', they will not realise that they are consciously creating manifesting limerence, or that these LOs are not 'objectively evocative', but rather, evocative to them because they complement them in a toxic way. Throughout the next few pages, we will cover why you are falling into limerence from a combined behavioural, psychological and spiritual perspective.

21. Meet Your Needs, Or Sabotage Every Aspect of Your Life

Much self-help material focuses on trying to make us less 'needy', promoting self-love and independence. The latter two attitudes are essential in living a purposeful, limerence-free life, but, not all needs can or should be 'healed out of'. While some must be overcome to escape from limerence and attract stable partners, must be met to keep us healthy, inspired and satisfied with life. The trick lies in discerning a). needs that are curated in response to trauma and are damaging, and b). needs that are real, primitive, and inescapable.

For example, it is unusual for an adult to feel the need to message their partner non-stop throughout the workday, and more abnormal for them to grow dysphoric when instant replies aren't granted. A 'need' of this nature is nearly always the result of mild to moderate childhood neglect, and should be treated as such and be overcome through targeted introspection. Raising children is one of life's most difficult tasks, and even the most diligent of parents fail to unwaveringly provide children with what they need. Perhaps one of your parents was forbidding and always busy with work, occasionally relaxing and drowning you in gifts and affection. A parental dynamic involving such a strong element of intermittent reward (see Chapter 31) primes you to seek similar patterns of reinforcement as an adult, because your brain associates those waves of attention with love. As romantic relationships are the best candidates for this intensity of bonding in adulthood, this type of upbringing can leave you drawn to flighty, capricious characters; after all, only unstable people who run hot-and-cold can (and will be driven to) intermittently reward you in this way.

Remember, as with all biological phenomena, all needs can be found on a spectrum ranging from those that are limiting and incompatible with healthy romance (such as our example above) to those that should be embraced as integral features of your personality. This latter category will englobe both a). deep, visceral cravings and b). the whimsical desiring of things that tickle our fancy. For example, you are gay, an obvious, irrefutable need of yours will be that your partner is the same gender as you; this core pillar of your nature should never be neglected. A more subtle example could be the desire to go on spontaneous adventures with your partner. This streak of rebelliousness and lust for life will be something snugly ingrained in your fixed values and needs, as well as reflected in your emotional intelligence and general passion for exploring the world.

Permit yourself to quench your thirst when it comes to your intrinsic needs, for sating these emotional, physical and spiritual requirements is essential for you to experience life **fully and expansively**. By shifting your awareness to them, your brain is telling you that you require something to promote your survival and happiness. If you fail to heed these warnings, you are not only heading towards *but are guaranteed* a limerent episode … if you are genetically capable of experiencing the state, that is.

22. Limerence Invariably Involves Unmet Needs

If you dislike that your current partner does not relate to you playfully and spontaneously, or take you up on your make-shift camping plans, this sense of 'lack' should be observed and respected; it is not something that psychotherapy, hypnosis or analytical introspection will free you from. You two are fundamentally a poor match, as you cannot meet each other's needs. While they may not be prone to strong infatuation, your partner will also have needs that are not being met and may display this by growing distant or seeming glum. Perhaps their genetic makeup renders them naturally passive and, furthermore, they were raised by tranquil, devoted parents who cherished long, slow meals together in the comfort of their own home. Adventures abroad that involve 'roughing it out' in cheap hostels to save money will be going against these core needs of theirs, which led to them desiring a wholesome, simple existence with you in the first place. While you will resend their 'dullness' and miss your wilder days with other partners, their needs will be being equally neglected and they will feel unsafe and unsatisfied.

If a limerence-prone person lets this type of **fundamental, glaring discrepancy** between their psychological needs and their lifestyle *go ignored*, they will be certain to run into a LO sooner or later. This man or woman will ooze red flag material left, right and centre, but will effortlessly reel them in as their teeth stay clenched to the bait like a *starving salmon*. Their keenness to embark on reckless road trips (and connect far too intensely and quickly) will set this repressed limerent's soul on fire, because they have been ravenous for so, so long.

We all must feed ourselves *emotionally and spiritually* to blossom as our true selves and get the most out of life; neglecting your needs will result in chronic resentment, a lack of fulfilment and stunted emotional growth. But, if you are prone to limerence, doing so is absolutely necessary and urgent. You must realise that if you live in discord with your innermost desires, you are effectively a ticking time bomb. Sooner or later, your brain will send a dose of chaos your way in a desperate, final attempt to get you to respect your needs.

Hopefully, that little vignette (involving our fictitious limerent) has served to show what can happen when you suppress aspects of your nature and allow the butterfly effect to work against you. Very quickly, a suboptimal life is created in front of you and you are left vulnerable, embittered and unfulfilled. Limerents are inquisitive, cerebral and daring people; I cannot stress how important acknowledging all of these needs of yours is when you are prone to limerence. Since we live in a society that prioritises productivity, the maintenance of an unemotional façade, and the ability to secure long-term, monogamous relationships, many of us fall into lives that are poor fits to our basal needs.

However, it is never too late to evolve from a situation that does not entirely serve you; it may just save your sanity or even your life. You are who you are, and cannot change what lights you up; do not live in a way that goes against the grain of your nature. You feeling happy, liberated and inspired is evolutionarily very important, as, in this state, we are better at hunting, foraging and reproducing. Therefore, we are <u>wired to be guided by desires</u>. Those that are reliably voiced to you as you pass through life should be honoured and met, as long as they do not harm others. Everything about your physiology tends towards disease, inflammation and general suboptimal functionality when any one of your core needs are ignored.

Take control of the steering wheel and create opportunities in your life that move you a little closer towards securing whatever feelings you treasure and enjoy. Until you do this, the primitive machinery of your limbic brain will look for **'twin flame' saviour figures** who make you feel better but who inevitably destroy your peace of mind, productivity and sanity.

23. Your Beliefs Create Your Reality

Do not fret; this book is not about to take a sharp turn and descend entirely into the metaphysical. However, it is an objective truth that your beliefs align you with everything that you can experience in this embodied existence. The amount of money you make, your level of fitness, your friendships, your romantic relationships and even whether or not people approach you in the street is the reflection_of your beliefs regarding yourself, others and the world.

American mystic Neville Goddard preached that when any belief or assumption is held in your mind, it inevitably hardens into reality. In this way, every element of your life in this time-space reality can be traced back to something you believe to be true about yourself, others or the world as a whole. People show up exactly as you imagine them, a phenomenon referred to as 'everyone is you pushed out' in the Goddard community. This is not to say that they always act how you want them to act, but rather, that they invariably act **how you believe** they can and will act (i.e. per your assumptions).

This line of thinking can be categorised as the Law of Assumption, and is a far superior belief system to the Law of Attraction which often misses the point. Many YouTubers and bloggers will be unamused with me for spilling the tea, but visualising attractive outcomes will get you nowhere if your identity and fundamental beliefs are not changing. The universe impartially slots you into situations that resonate with your specific frequency, aligning you with things that confirm who you are, not who you *want* to be. Forget karma, begging for your 'specific person' or crafting up dream boards of Ferraris, this new age spirituality is futile if you are not doing transformative work alongside it.

Remember, leaders in those fields and their marketing teams do just about everything possible to keep you addicted to them. They know that selling you mind-numbing, pain-alleviating candyfloss dreams will help you feel a little better about your current situation but *will* never cure you, hence you will become dependent on their services and content. For this reason, they resist imparting to you the only 'spiritual' truth out there, which is that we do not get what we deserve, what we would really like, or what our lovely grandmother visualises us with. **We get more of who we are**, and who we 'feel' ourselves to be on a deep level. Given reality is an elastic, malleable playground, it goes without saying that you can be financially independent and live on the beach in Argentina, and you can meet the absolute love of your life and leave limerence behind. However, someone who believes that the world is unjust and who guards intense resentment for anyone who is in a solid relationship, trying to impress their subconscious mind with the concept of a 'soulmate' entering their life will be fruitless. Instead, they must unravel the undesirable wirings behind their belief system regarding romance and change who they feel they are; the world will shifts in accordance, as it always bears witness to such internal changes.

24. Be Careful What You Assume

The Law of Assumption undeniably and irrevocably governs this entire universe with no exceptions or inconsistencies. Let me illustrate its workings with three examples that should cajole you towards seeing just how your limerence habit is the result of your thinking patterns, assumptions and, hence, identity:

- **The Draining Friend**: Imagine you have a troublesome, bitter friend who talks about you behind your back, constantly tries to embarrass you and scoffs at anything that you are proud of. This situation has arisen because a). on some subconscious level, you do not believe that you are worth more than this, and b). you two share some limiting beliefs about the world resulting in both of you occupying a shared space of emotional disarray. The fact that you have stayed in this platonic relationship (and attracted it in the first place) confirms that this friend's way of treating you resonates with your own frequency. Perhaps you both feel cheated by society and frustrated at not having achieved your goals; in response, your friend grows nasty and tries to establish a power dynamic over you, while you assume a position of learned helplessness and tolerate low-level trauma from them because *receiving any attention is worth it*. If you decided to make tomorrow a different day, challenged limiting beliefs about how life is 'unfair', switched from a scarcity mindset towards one of abundance and pursued intriguing hobbies, you would no longer feel so vulnerable or dependent on them. By not needing their suboptimal attention, they would no longer get their ego bowed down to by you and would be repulsed by the situation; narcissists do not get anything from people with healthy, functional boundaries and a sense of purpose. The result would be both of your paths bifurcating cleanly and effortlessly and them sailing out of your life, as you can only experience what you are not a vibrational match for.

- **The 'Red Pill' Subscriber:** Now, we are going to consider a hypothetical example of the power of the Law in the realm of romance. Let's imagine a man who has grown up believing that women are fickle, untrustworthy and superficial. A deep part of him yearns for a success-driven and loyal girlfriend, but his baseline stance towards dating is one of resentfulness and despair; he cannot seem to pique and keep the attention of a suitable woman, instead attracting beautiful but mentally-vacant individuals who waste his time. Unaware that he is manifesting these outcomes through his limiting beliefs, he takes to the internet and posts on forums about how 'women are only a nuisance' and that 'heterosexual men are better off focusing on work and friendship'.

Unsurprisingly, in such 'echo chambers' you are rewarded for speaking out by others with the same unhealed psychological wounds as you, so this belief system of his pertaining to women and romance is only strengthened with ferocity over the years. What he does not realise is that, if he spent two hours considering how skewed and embittered the lens through which he is viewing the world is, he would shift himself into a new reality and radiate the energy that strong, proud, interesting women want and need from a partner. He currently deals with dull, transient flings, because, by vibrationally screaming to the world that "women are not equal to men", he can *only* experience women who also believe this to be true, who inevitably come along with an array of traits conducive to this passive, jaded stance towards life. In this situation, he could become the protagonist of his own story and create the exact life that he wants by simply questioning and changing the flawed beliefs that he defends and identifies with. One simple, effective way for this man to do this would be by remembering that his mother is also a woman, and most likely one he adores and respects who boasts a set of wonderful qualities.

- **The Bright, Tortured Limerent**: Finally, we are going to look at how beliefs can align us with *limerence* specifically. I have purposefully created a complex example that can easily be extrapolated from, to allow you to dig deep and ascertain which assumptions of *yours* are occupying a place of prominence in your limerence habit.

Let me introduce our subject, Ciara. She is an effusive, likeable thirty-year-old woman with a sharp sense of humour and a large circle of equally entertaining friends. In terms of her career, her health and her relationships with her friends and family, she is immensely satisfied and feels that she is 'a whiz at life'. What seems to be elusive and out of her reach, however, is a truly deep, intimate romantic relationship. She has dated several people, but has always ended up pushing her partner away due to finding the relationship too stable, predictable and lacking in magic. What she craves profoundly is sitting and talking about **surreal, abstract concepts** and sharing the dreams that set her soul on fire with a special someone.

Once every two years or so, she does come across someone who shares her mental wavelength and engages in this form of sublime connection with her. Her voracious appetite for enmeshment with these people has landed her in some incredibly strong infatuations, and the problem is that they are always complex, tortured and difficult individuals. Each time, she's instantly overcome with the sensation that they are meant for her, and romanticises this feeling as <u>evidence for a 'twin flame bond'</u> rather than questioning the root cause of her **psychological reactivity** to them. Despite being overwhelmingly exciting, these connections never, ever advance into anything more than a few weeks of mutual brain-picking, and Ciara always ends up losing touch with them because they do not act like other people she knows. They detach from her as quickly as they initially took to her, and compliments and Tuesday night star-gazing transitions into radio silence. Only left with the photos that they took together, she tries to decipher a). why these adults run so hot and cold and b). what is spurring her on to engage with them, over and over again.

Do you see some of yourself in Ciara? She is actively aligning with limerence, despite being independent, feisty and *actively cognizant* that her experience of love is too strong and unsustainable to ever equate to any form of permanence. Referring back at Chapter 21, she is harbouring unmet needs regarding a). general romantic intimacy and b). expressing herself verbally and being truly 'seen'. While the latter unmet need is perfectly normal and cannot be 'healed out of' (those of us who are not aromantic will sometimes crave romantic companionship), her ineffably strong desire to be **protected and enshrouded** by the energy of her LOs is not healthy and is related to category problematic unmet needs that she has developed over time.

Ciara experiences a strong yearning for an overwhelming form of intimacy that she is unlikely to receive from anyone; toddles who are continuously coddled by their primary caregivers are protected, reaffirmed and endorsed in this way, but adults are not. She deals with this abnormal, trauma-stemming need because she does not experience enough <u>sublime, euphoric connection</u> with herself or anyone else in her life. She is clearly complex and intelligent, requiring a good amount of mental stimulation and real recognition for who she is, as a <u>sparkly, multi-faceted</u> being living an embodied existence. Years of not receiving even a sliver of what she emotionally needs have resulted in her suffering greatly, and undergoing continuous small-scale traumas. Her entire being is shouting at her to grant herself at least *some* of what she needs.

In order to decrease her ache for intimacy, protection and constant reinforcement from LOs who provide her with deep conversations but will never commit, she must meet these needs elsewhere. This will involve her committing to showing up in life as **the most authentic version of herself** possible; regardless of how daunting it feels, this woman needs to imagine life as a dream, decide what she would do and say if it were, and then apply that to real life.

Moreover, she will need to express herself and use fluid, evocative language as often as possible, as her tendency to indiscriminately sentimentalise all intimate verbal exchanges indicates that self-expression enlivens her beyond belief. Perhaps a blog, a YouTube channel or becoming a motivational speaker would bring her the affirming feeling of 'having an audience' that she loves so much when alone with a LO. So far, we have not touched on the **assumptions and beliefs**, only needs; however, you already know that these different takes on limerence are inextricably intertwined. Altering your assumptions and, hence, your self-esteem is an absolute prerequisite to meeting your needs; committing to *doggedly pursuing* the earthly feelings that you love regardless of what aspects of your former life may dissolve away is contingent on you knowing that amazing, healthily euphoric, limerent-free times lie ahead of you. When you are enticed by what emotional freedom will entail and (crucially) you trust in your innate ability to edge yourself towards it, you have successfully flipped your belief systems; they are now tuned away from corroborating the presence of pre-existing trauma and towards manifesting you your dreams.

I hope this final example has allowed you to see the distinct but overlapping roles that a). belief systems and b). unmet needs play in generating limerence. When you are unaware that limerence is a reflection of you, these psychological areas of weakness will nucleate into the various elements of the limerent experience. However, the day that you truly assimilate the concept that you are in control, everything changes. Today can and should be that day for you; in Chapter 28, you will learn how to scientifically and precisely communicate with your subconscious mind to eradicate unhelpful assumptions/beliefs and instil new ones.

25. From Genetics to The Numinous

Now that we have analysed the makeup of limerence from different angles, I would like to draw your attention to the fact that we are often force-fed and expected to swallow a false dichotomy between science and spirituality. The two are far from mutually exclusive and irreconcilable; neuroscience and psychology not only vouch for but also substantiate the view of the world that I have described in the previous chapter. Everyone who has become a billionaire, gained academic prestige or overcome a disorder like limerence has one thing in common: each one came to realise that ideas **held in their subconscious mind** were creating their entire life, in all its good and bad aspects, and decided to start consciously creating favourable outcomes.

We have covered the neurobiological correlates of the state and we know that thinking methodically and scientifically is essential in obtaining clarity and closure. However, considering limerence in terms of spirituality and interpersonal energetic dynamics is the most effective way to tweak your identity and become limerence-immune. Of course, the scientific basis of you acting distinctly, entertaining different desires and being drawn to different people is the altered expression of the genes that encode proteins important to neurotransmission (which, in turn, results in altered neuronal pathways and differential communication between brain regions).

As progressive neuroscientists like Dr Joe Dispenza communicate, visualising and mentally stepping into a superior version of yourself results in epigenetic mechanisms being activated, consequent alterations in gene expression and a transformed brain and mentality. Epigenetics describes the interplay between your genetics and environmental factors, and such cascades are occurring in your brain all the time; when you learn a new skill and start to feel differently about the world or you experience years of chronic stress, your epigenome and, hence, the proteins expressed in your brain, are being selectively tweaked. Considering this alone indicates that great potential lies in studying spirituality through a biological lens – and, importantly, that spiritual techniques and attitudes are capable of altering your biology and freeing you from states like limerence.

Furthermore, this universe that we inhabit appears to be governed by peculiar forces and laws, that even quantum physics cannot come close to deciphering. Even the most analytical of us occasionally find ourselves stumped by unexpected synchronicities far too uncanny to be fully explained by logic. Spirituality is an invaluable tool when dealing with the deep, rich emotions of limerence and the ebbs and flows of life in general, and I highly suggest that you approach it playfully and incorporate it into your stance towards reality. Our monkey brains fall short of omniscience, so we do not know if what we categorise as 'spiritual happenings' are a). wild emergent phenomena with elusive but scientifically-explicable roots or b). downright magic, but do not let this worry you. Learn to *lean into the magic* and see how it complements, rather than threatens, all of the important neurobiological truths that we have covered.

26. What Thoughts Do You Have About Love?

Now, we are going to consider the different components of a **belief system**, since these are what the Law of Assumption states are bound to materialise in your life. Your belief system regarding romance neatly encloses all of the feelings, thoughts, intuitions and hunches that are instantly stirred up when you consider the topic of 'love'. We are going to explore just how your thinking patterns dictate whether or not you, as a limerence-prone person, end up actually attracting and aligning with the suboptimal, illusory form of love that limerence is. The term **'belief'** refers to the deeply ingrained *acceptance* that something is true (even in the absence of proof), and beliefs generate a string of **thoughts** concerning that particular topic. As intelligent sentient beings, we believe our thoughts, perceiving them as belonging to our innermost intuition.

First and foremost, I want you to truly understand what a **thought** is, and what positive and negative implications stem from treating thoughts as 'perfect indications' of what is happening in this reality. Nearly every single person on this planet identifies with and trusts their thoughts and emotions as if they are objective facts. However, I am here to tell you that they are not, and that rejecting the primitive, convincing arguments that your brain transmits to you about your inability to overcome limerence will immunise you from it.

The truth is that 'thought' can be almost considered a sensory modality (i.e. a sense), just as smell, touch and hearing are; we perceive a <u>stimulus</u> in our surroundings and neural connections orchestrate a <u>response</u> to that stimulus (e.g. we bat a fly away from our face, or interject when someone addresses us rudely), in addition to <u>generating thoughts</u>. Many psychologists tell their patients that their negative *thinking* patterns give rise to negative *emotions*; this is often true, but occasionally an oversimplification.

As with everything pertaining to neuroscience, clean causal relationships are rare due to the computational complexity of the brain. Therefore, we cannot state that 'thoughts cause emotions, and never the other way around'; for example, while the raw emotional state induced in you by the death of a relative is the result of the thoughts you experienced upon hearing the horrible news, those same emotions will make you more likely to experience more negative thoughts for weeks. In this way, we see an intricate relationship and *feedback loop* between thoughts and emotions; strong emotions do arise from thoughts, but *also* provide your brain with some context through which to view the world. This means that they sometimes <u>influence future thoughts</u>. Another example: if your brother shouts at you and you two argue pettily for hours (in a way that upsets you), you will **experience negative thoughts** and proverbially roll your eyes if he later asks you to do him a favour.

With the **bidirectional relationship** between thoughts and emotions acknowledged, we are going to move on and look at <u>one side</u> of it: when emotions *can* be considered the output effect (i.e. the consequence) of thoughts, which are the smallest unit of a belief system.

Just as we can walk into the kitchen, have our appetite whetted by the aroma of garlic and onion and start to want some dinner, we may feel uncomfortable at the dentist's, deal with intrusive thoughts about the steely object approaching our mouth and consequently be seized by adrenaline and panic. Both of these examples involve your brain processing an external stimulus and inducing a reaction; just as the olfactory centres in your brain orchestrate your ability to 'smell', your cortex generates 'thoughts' that are reflective of the integration of <u>all of the sensory components</u> of what you are experiencing.

Due to the **great interconnectivity** between the brain regions involved in thought production, thoughts are also always greatly influenced by your past experiences and beliefs (in addition to the emotional state that you are already in, as we have seen with our preceding examples). Intrusive dental procedures trigger instinctive fear through amygdala-centred circuits in everyone, because we are all primed to fear being contained in a seat while unfamiliar people approach our faces with odd 'weapons'. However, if you are someone who underwent a very painful, unexpected tooth extraction as a young child, you are more likely to feel negatively about the experience than a young member of the Royal Family who has only ever received the most gentle, attentive dental care.

By talking about emotions as an <u>emergent phenomenon created by thoughts</u>, which are in turn influenced by our autobiographical memories, I am describing aspects of the human experience that you will already be familiar with. Aspects that are often described with quotes like 'our perception is clouded by our past', 'adults cannot experience *things as innocently* as children' or 'the brain utilises emotionally-evocative memories to place new sensations and experiences in context'.

Things get a little more complicated when we remember that our thoughts, which collectively form our 'perception' of any given situation, are *not* flawlessly-accurate, truth-bearing messengers. They are the result of the brain's miraculous, but ultimately highly imperfect, way of comprehending input from sensory receptors that scan the world around it <u>based on past experiences</u>. This constant integration of the 'past and present' is often extremely useful, saving our lives, but can also be very detrimental and result in conditions like limerence (when we start to believe that a beautiful relationship is out of our reach), phobias and neurosis. A good example of this risk-averse vigilance going awry would be a someone ritualistically avoiding parks and running away from puppies, just because their father dislikes dogs and told her that they were all dangerous when she was a child.

Her brain has erroneously grouped dogs together as a trigger stimulus, based on her dad's narrative; whether they be gentle, foreboding, fluffy or teacup-sized, they terrify her and experiencing them sets off a train of thoughts that kick her autonomic nervous system into action (thanks to amygdaloid neurons communicating with the hypothalamus). Seeing a small Pug generates an energy-taxing, upsetting and embarrassing response in her that burdens her with cognitive load and renders her more tired for the rest of the day… all without promoting her survival, for there was no real risk. Communication between neurons in her brain that are **interconnected** with those that *encode memories* of her anti-canine indoctrination (thanks, dad) generate thoughts about dogs that are scary and untrue.

At this point, it must be pointed out that the opposite adaptation can, and does, occur, having tragic effects in the more dangerous domains of life. A child who is raised in a sheltered, crime-free Cornish village and denied use of the internet may end up in a sticky situation when they first visit a big city, having only ever socialised with the same trusty family friends and schoolmates for sixteen years. When they realise that certain people are ill-intentioned, prepared to lie about others to get ahead socially, or that someone who acts like a friend on a night out and hugs them might be doing so just to snatch their iPhone, they suffer reality collapse.

This type of 'shock' can manifest itself in dissociative anxiety symptoms and denial, as the person subconsciously decides to reject this new information rather than accepting that the **reality paradigm** that they believed to be true as a child is wholly unrealistic. Reality collapse similarly occurs when people raised by intolerant and/or sanctimonious families realise that they are gay. Therapy and effective introspection work wonders in allowing your brain to re-process emotional trauma of this nature, and weave all that you know into one big *reality model* that feels welcoming rather than uninhabitable.

Now, we are summing up what we have covered on **the role that thoughts play** in generating emotions. Humans are certainly incredibly intellectual and perceptive animals; your ability to notice thoughts, clearly isolate them and react to them is priceless and pertinent to your survival. If you were not capable of this, you would be as naïve as our recent example, and unable to pick up on a malevolent, aggressive aura and distance yourself before a disaster. You would be equally incapable of recognising **gratifying things in life** that make you happy and thinking 'oh yes, this is something I am going to continue doing!'. However, in the context of an obsessional, pathological 'dead-end' like limerence, we see the dark sides of these mechanisms in place.

Thoughts, and the emotions that follow, are inextricably connected with your bank of memories and the belief systems that you have curated over the years. This can go very wrong when you are feeding yourself with a negative mental diet, subscribing to skewed beliefs and assuming the stance of a 'victim of love' who will never again taste emotional freedom.

27. Question Your Thoughts, Challenge Your Established Belief Systems

You have experienced limerence; it thus will not cost you much imaginal power to intuit that the thoughts produced by your limerent brain, and hence the lenses through which you view the world, are more tainted by limiting beliefs than those of the average person.

For someone married who has become limerent for the first time, it may be tempting to remain convinced that their LO is the most enlivening, admirable person alive, and that no real relationship, whether with their spouse or their friends, will ever emotionally sate them again. For a limerent who starts to experience obsessive crushes as a teenager, fights unrequited love in vain as an adult and sees everyone around them in mutual relationships while they ideate suicide over someone who barely sends them regular text messages, it might seem 'prudent' to come to terms with the fact that normal love is impossibly out of reach. But, negative mental frameworks are neither **true depictions of reality** nor **fixed**; neuroplasticity is always at work, and will work in your favour once you learn to grab the wheel with resolution and start amending them.

By buying into a). your feelings of dread about romance and b). your primitive cravings for someone to meet your unmet needs (rather than meeting them yourself), you are not giving yourself a chance to shine and be independent. You attract exactly the outcome that is the sum of those beliefs, intuitions and thoughts, which is more LOs; you believe that **romantic contentedness** is impossible for you, but not that it is impossible for you *to click* with or attract people, and these exact assumptions are reflected in your life. You get to know people who 'glimmer', but you can't ever quite catch them. You end up riding highs and lows based on whether or not they are giving you attention.

The law of mirroring governs this entire universe, and similar things coalesce together effortlessly. Thoughts are followed by like thoughts, and you will always draw people and outcomes towards you like a powerful magnet. The wonderful news is that, just as changing the metal composition of a magnet will change its power, learning to question your thoughts and intrinsic beliefs will send you on the trajectory of attracting wildly different things.

As if by magic, you will no longer find the same LOs appealing, because they will not resonate with you by meeting your unmet needs or confirming one of your existing beliefs. People of their nature will dissolve away in the periphery, and real partners who make you excited, thrilled and contented, rather than manic, overwhelmed and depressed, will take centre stage. And, if you are already in a relationship, you will be well-poised to re-enter a state of harmony and alignment with your partner; **the insanity will be over**.

28. How to Practically Programme Your Subconscious Mind With Different Beliefs

Fortunately, as we have brushed over in former chapters (particularly when we looked at the examples of how the Law of Assumption contributes to limerence) we can wake up to the fact that we are constantly manifesting experiences and people into our lives and learn to use this law **intentionally and skilfully**. The psychological basis of this lies in altering the beliefs and ideas that you subconsciously subscribe to, as what you consider true on an intuitive level is always reflected directly into this physical realm (in the form of people, prosperity, opportunities, health and problems). In other words, believe something and you will be shown confirmation of this belief.

Henry Ford: *"whether you think you can, or you think you can't – you're right."*

See your subconscious mind as a printer, and the 3D existence that you experience as the piece of paper that emerges. A mere print out of computer information, it just 'is', untouched by and neutral to human morality, *your* goals or what you would like to experience. It does not matter how much you desire an outcome in life – until you **become the version of yourself** who believes that s/he deserves it and can have it, you will not be operating in a way that permits that thing to enter your reality.

Fortunately, you do not need to be one hundred percent convicted that you are 'guaranteed to receive' what you wish for to align with it, although unwavering faith is potent and bound to speed up the timeline for you. You just need to view yourself as someone who *can* receive it; this, as I, and many others, have come to see, really comes down to a 'yes' or 'no' answer. Either you think something is possible for you, or you don't.

A powerful way to gauge whether you need to work on certain beliefs is to consider yourself receiving what you want, and identify how you feel – whether you are imbued with fear and disbelief or quite, hopeful excitement. Naturally, we have all been inculcated with different ideas since childhood, lived very different lives and encountered different struggles, so what we deem 'possible' will sit in consonance with these multifarious factors. Someone may be accomplished, successful and with a real eye for detail, yet struggle with the realm of romantic relationships and host many beliefs regarding their inability to get anyone's attention in a non-platonic way. This person will automatically 'feel' that they're capable of putting in all-nighters to finish a novel that they are writing, because they have proved to themselves countless times that they are proficient at both committing to and *seeing through such goals*.

However, when asked to imagine themself having a partner who they genuinely feel inspired to say "I love you" to, knowing that they have met someone truly matched to them, the same person might find that this feels like a distant pipe dream – or, if accustomed to and accepting of their 'inability' to attract such outcomes, may even laugh off the idea as implausible and surreal. If very self-aware, someone in this position may identify this resistance of theirs as a sign that they need to pattern their mind with new concepts and beliefs until the idea of booking a Valentine's Day reservation/planning a weekend getaway with a future partner seems pleasant but natural… almost tangible. In contrast, another person might inherently 'know' that they are beautiful, but believe that the opposite sex is impossible to read and thus impossible to connect with, rendering them closed-off, critical, untrusting, and unknowingly trapped in a cycle of half-hearted, unsatisfying connections.

When their friends suggest that they experiment with dating apps, or ask a real-life acquaintance out, someone in this position might roll their eyes, well aware that they *can* conjure up a **generic, semi-pleasing connection** whenever they feel like doing so. What would tug at this person's emotions a little more, however, would be imagining themself in a committed relationship and making a scrapbook for their partner's birthday. Imagining a scene of this nature may stir up deep resentment and pain, indicative of how impossible they feel that *meaningful* romance is for them.

Here lies the boundary between what this person deems natural for them and what they struggle to currently imagine themselves aligning with, and right behind this is a web of deeply ingrained beliefs that are generating these assumptions. Rather than being a melancholy revelation that 'real love will forever remain elusive', the sombre pain that this person might feel upon reflecting should **encourage them to push themselves** and break through to a new level of life – to do whatever it takes to allow novel things to flow into their reality. There is nothing to lose in a situation like this, and everything to gain; with the correct attitude, this person is more than capable of rapidly altering their beliefs, their self-identity and, in turn, their love life.

It is extremely important to elucidate *your own* points of resistance by imaging yourself in a plethora of different situations and considering which feel normal, and which feel ridiculously out of reach. This person here does not need to work on their self-esteem, nor necessarily on 'trusting people' in general if they have healthy, happy friendships. What they really need to do is **re-sculpt their beliefs** about truly fulfilling potential romantic partners and the level of connection that they, as an individual, are capable of securing with these individuals. Currently, their beliefs are counterproductive and, despite feeling like 'objective truths' and logical deductions given their life experience thus far, are not, for **your reality overwhelmingly reflects your beliefs**, *rather than* the other way around.

When you consider all of your own romantic experiences (whether stints of requited or unrequited love), you will see just how precisely and uncannily a belief of this nature is translated into your life until it is sorted out. You will definitely, at this point, be able to deduce which ideas you are currently hosting about yourself, your relationship with other human beings and the way romance should/can work have snowballed to land you in limerence. It is likely that a lot of you reading this, however, will be dealing with problematic beliefs that are much more subtle than our aforementioned examples. I also realise, and have confirmed to me on a weekly basis from interesting emails I receive from readers of my content, that the chaos that limerence subjects a lot of you to is **in clear juxtaposition** with the other facets of your life. Most of you are accomplished, empathetic, proactive individuals who wonder how on earth the mental framework that rewards you with continuous dividends in so many areas of your life has simultaneously primed you for limerence. Whether you have only known limerence, or these feelings have unexpectedly hit you for the first time at a later age, you will most likely indignantly ponder how/why you can be composed, stoic and logical when it comes to different platonic and family matters, yet find yourself craving 'scraps' from a character in your life who is bizarrely able to determine your mood for the entirety of the day.

"But What If I Think My Belief Systems Are Fine? If I'm Successful In So Many Areas of Life, How Do I Know What to Change?"

Worry not, for this confusion is perfectly normal. A). Your beliefs regarding different areas of life can (and normally do) vary remarkably, and b). we are often poor at objectively gauging what we really feel/believe before the importance of doing so is brought to our attention. Someone could, for example, believe they were highly lucky and capable of peak performance, which would cajole them towards entering lots of competitions, pushing themselves at work, and being receptive to professional opportunities that might come their way. The same person may, however, have a real complex with food and struggle to make peace with their healthy body weight. Their beliefs/assumptions about their ability to a). pull off a really good presentation despite having prepared at the last minute and b). be happy on holiday with their friends on the beach will, unfortunately, be diametrically opposed.

Hopefully, this example will stimulate you to peer *behind* the positive, fruitful beliefs that you have successfully instilled into your mind over the span of your life, and critically identify which **equally-influential but negative** ones you also subscribe to and are being controlled by.

Suspend Your Disbelief: To Get Different Results In Life, We Must Try Different Things

If all this talk of 'beliefs' still sounds very esoteric to you, do not worry – all will be clear after we consider a few more examples and look at the techniques that will yield you quantifiable, visible results. You will slowly but surely grasp how your thinking has enabled you to not only tolerate the nightmarish phenomenon that is limerence, but actually become somewhat addicted to it and wonder whether it could promise you your most authentic reality. The specific limerent neural makeup that we have discussed in previous chapters is necessary to feel that initial 'jolt' of adrenaline, and to consequently obsess over the same person (i.e. set of stimuli) and become so deeply depressed, but sustained limerence is only possible when your beliefs about yourself/others/what you can and should expect from love are suboptimal. This should come as fantastic news; this, along with other psychological components of limerence including unmet needs, can be changed in *anyone* who is willing to tolerate initial discomfort and have faith in their brain's ability to ***neatly and magnificently*** mend itself.

Beliefs are behind everything; no person on this planet is immune to the fact that their beliefs are constantly creating their reality. Anyone who has achieved things that they are delighted with in a sustained way has done so while watching the mental conversations that they have with themselves on a daily basis. Some individuals are very blessed and find that this comes to them naturally; without much prompting, they come to soberly, irrefutably see that no momentum builds up in their mind without materialising/having its effect on their life, in due course. Then, they tentatively experiment with changing the direction of some of their thoughts, only to find proof, time in and time out, that this sets new things into motion that they previously never used to experience.

Others have parents with unusual levels of emotional intelligence, who knew exactly how to teach them how to manage their own psychology from a young age and counter intrusive thoughts. Most of us, however, have to commit to learning the ropes ourselves, until optimising our headspace becomes second nature and we can whip out the pruning shears and **excise unwanted beliefs** with seamless precision when we first notice them rearing their heads.

More Examples of Beliefs In Action

Continuing with our examples to prompt your brain to come to conclusions about your *own* belief systems, let's imagine that you are someone who is relatively happy with their academic/professional/financial success, enthused about a lot of interesting topics and good at adhering to a fun and rewarding exercise routine. Despite being self-assured most of the time, however, you have always yearned for an extremely deep, intimate connection with someone who understands the complexities of your mind inside-out. You consider yourself attractive and intelligent, so do not struggle to strike up connections and get to know people. However, your issue is that very few people resonate with you on a romantic level, and when they do, there seems to be *resistance*.

You seem to repel these people just as the connection properly starts to bloom, and cannot comprehend why – it is like your emotional poise goes out of the window. Despite trying to hide it, you become insecure, self-critical and focused on the goal (a magical relationship with this person and the security and euphoria that you believe that will bring you) and this **energy inevitably infiltrates** your online and real-life communication with them. Over the span of a few weeks, you cease to be the playful, relaxed individual who they were initially attracted to, and who you truly *are*, and assume a state that renders you a poor fit for a healthy relationship with them or anyone. This elicits unpleasant responses from the person in question, and triggers their detachment from their connection with you. Which, as you are forced to accept, has been nothing more than at transient spark; once again, love has somehow eluded you.

Consequently, you are left heartbroken, thinking "I knew it – the people I like lose interest once they see the real me… this is the last time I get my hopes up." However, while this conclusion (and these beliefs) may feel like **a logical inference** to take away from what you have so far experienced in life, you are missing the point that you are the architect of your reality. **You have unknowingly unstilled** these beliefs into your subconscious mind and, unaware of their power, have allowed them to grow, resulting in them hardening into reality and profoundly influencing your behaviour. And, consequently, in you seeing more and more 'proof' of them.

Unfortunately, the fact that our beliefs dictate our entire lives leads us to erroneously conclude that they are undeniably true judgments that we have prudently made – we believe that our beliefs are indicative of the *real status of reality*, when the truth is that this works the other way around for the most part.

You see, your beliefs **powerfully permeate and dictate** your mood, energy, actions and communication, and are, whether you choose to view this neuroscientifically, psychologically or spiritually, the root of all mental afflictions. In this example, it is your beliefs that are actually causing the premature, painful curtailment of these budding romantic connections. An easily identifiable **umbrella belief** is to blame for all your misery, and changing it would provoke a delightful one hundred and eighty degree shift in your life. Transforming the single belief that "special people are hard to come by – it is my job to secure a connection before it slips away" would stop you a). becoming nervous and clingy, b). this being reflected undesirably in your behaviour, text messages and presence, and c). deterring potential partners who you could, in actual fact, live out mentally stimulating, fulfilling relationships with while in the right receptive, relaxed, abundant headspace.

If you are reading this and are married or in a **serious, committed relationship**, that does not mean that you are exempt from having to control your beliefs about yourself/romance/others. All of this information applies to you just as much as it does to single, young limerents who are finding their way in life and navigating romantic feelings for the first time. It will also be just as crucial to your recovery from limerence. It is very likely that your beliefs about your partner, yourself and your worthiness of their love, are generally positive; when it comes to your LO, however, a multitude of beliefs regarding how they are more powerful than you, how you need their energy in your life and how embarrassing the whole situation is proving is playing a causal role in keeping you trapped in limerence.

Your unmet needs naturally come into this, too, being another pillar that must be attended to in order to become limerence immune; you erroneously <u>believe</u> that you can only feel enlivened, authentic and truly understood <u>with this person</u>. In reality, making small, consistent changes (or drastic actions, if you can) to your lifestyle, the people you mix with and the things you do will provide you with exactly what you are looking for and stop you being attracted to these LOs; actively taking action in this way while in this depressive headspace, however, will be contingent on having *faith in your ability* to meet your own needs. That, itself, is a belief that you need to plant and encourage to spread its roots, isn't it?

Imprinting Your Subconscious With Renewed Beliefs Pays Dividends, Permanently

At this point, it should now be crystal clear just how devastating the wrong thoughts and beliefs can be, encroaching on all aspects of your life (and even determining your ability to recover from limerence). Fortunately, establishing the right overarching belief systems will allow you to receive things, connections, opportunities and general abundance more magnificent than you can currently even envisage. You see, just like money invested in shares with high returns, the rewards yielded from beliefs that actually serve you compound over time… tremendously so.

On a practical level, how do we go about altering our belief systems? In order to leave behind problematic psychological frameworks, you must a). ascertain what limiting beliefs you have that pertain to yourself, your value, how people treat you and how romance should, and can, work and b). assimilate new ideas and beliefs that counter these **until your brain generates** new pathways and you intuit, feel and wholeheartedly believe them to be true. In the second part of this chapter, we will look at some infallible techniques that will enable you to imprint your subconscious mind while it is most receptive; these work for anyone when carried out diligently, regardless of how stubborn and deep-rooted you think some of your beliefs may be.

Before we delve into how to practically rewire your subconscious mind, we are going to consider a final example to cast light on why changing your **assumptions** is not only important, but crucial, for saying goodbye to limerence once and for all. Imagine you are a serial limerent who falls for LOs who are callous, sharp but authoritative in a way that is irresistible to you. To a certain extent, preferences *are* innate and reflective of your makeup, so you would not necessarily need to try and escape your primitive desire to date someone who is proud, independent and more dominant than you and settle for soft partners who do not sparkle to you at all. However, what you *would* need to do would be to alter your inner wirings so that you are no longer a fit for (or attracted to) someone who subjects you to cruel, unpredictable behaviour.

Consider the sheer enormity of the population, or even of the city or town that you live in; many people will exude the confident characteristics that you like but will also have functional boundaries, sharp communication skills and know better than to play with people's emotions by 'half-bonding' with them. These are the people that you, in this hypothetical example, should be dating, rather than the elusive LOs who possess some **hyper-magnified, damaging variants** of these traits and who you currently see as 'saviours'. Sure, hyper-aloof LOs lure you in because of your thus far untreated psychological points of vulnerability, but you can absolutely date someone whose independent nature thrills you but who can, to boot, actually fall in love with you and commit to you. You are in no way limited to LOs who orbit you, occasionally reaching out but ultimately lacking sincere interest in living out a real, requited chapter with you… unless you allow yourself to harbour beliefs that limit you to this expression of human connection.

I hope that you have found a shred of relatability in some of the examples I have presented you with in this section. However, even if none of them apply to your life experience and/or feelings towards LOs, I trust that they will have served to plant a seed in your mind that will now start flourishing on its own – **the crystallised realisation** that you are in full control of your own reality, and that, even though it feels tempting to drift through life, conclude things from your experiences and then adhere firmly to stances and positions concerning what is possible, you are infinitely limiting yourself and **fettering your potential** to live sublimely if you do so. No negative belief should ever lie unchallenged.

The Two Best Techniques to Develop New Beliefs (And Supplant Old Ones)

The techniques we are now going to look at all have one thing in common: they need to be carried out when you are in a deep state of relaxation, starting from 15-30 minutes before you fall asleep. In this state of relaxed wakefulness, the brain produces what are referred to as 'Alpha waves' (7.5-14 Hz) and the subconscious mind is very impressionable. During this window of time, **reprogramming of beliefs** is highly effective. Your goal with all of these techniques is to actively conjure up feelings/enter a different emotional state. They are all essentially, therefore, the means to the same end – to feel differently about whatever it is that you are addressing, before drifting off to sleep in this desirable state. This is the single most effective method to lay down new beliefs, and/or override ones that are not serving you.

Just to clarify, you should never let negative momentum grow when you are applying these techniques; don't think about how 'you are changing unwanted beliefs', or pay them any mind. Instead, just ascertain what the *opposite* beliefs are – which ones you want to adopt/replace them with– and focus on fostering those. Anything that you feel while in the Alpha state will start being instilled into your subconscious mind, because your brain will deem it to be real life experience. Therefore, great potential lies in transforming all aspects of your life with these techniques – I hope you continue to experiment with them once you have recovered entirely from limerence, for they will also improve your financial situation, health, physique, friendships, opportunities and just about anything else you can imagine.

The **creative power of your subconscious mind** is a force to be reckoned with – as well as influencing your physiological functions (heart rate, digestion, blood pressure), your brain's subconscious intrinsic activity (i.e. its activity at rest) also acts as a gatekeeper to modulate how your brain lays down memories, the emotional spectrum you experience on a day-to-day basis, how keen you are to take risks that offer future rewards, and which goals you are moving towards. Therefore, it is no exaggeration to say that your happiness and success depend heavily on you employing techniques to regulate your subconscious mind, particularly when you are capable of the type of obsessionality and the **rich emotional gamut** that facilitate the development of states like limerence.

I will also add a disclaimer that these techniques are by no means my own invention; the effectiveness of communicating with the subconscious mind when it is most receptive is established and unchallenged. The work of countless wonderful, forward-thinking psychologists, neuroscientists, doctors and New Age leaders have come to the same conclusion: all physical and mental afflictions can be traced, to some degree, to the subconscious mind. In the References section at the end of this book, I will add some further reading for those of you who are interested in exploring different elaborations of on these ideas. If, however, you simply wish to extricate yourself from the pain of limerence and return to a stable, functional, inspired state, there is no need to consume any of this additional content. You will achieve full recovery just by earnestly and optimistically engaging with these techniques. They all start to work immediately, and, when adhered to, will transform your beliefs in a serious, long-lasting way after around four-twelve weeks.

Just like every project worth starting, this process will require diligence and commitment. Soon after starting this self-work, you will start to feel renewed and generally better– the seeds that you are planting will already be sprouting. Your mood will be more stable and your outlook on life refreshed. It is crucial, however, that you *still* religiously stick to your chosen regimen after the onset of this emotional upswing; to alter your deep-rooted beliefs about love/yourself/others in the profound, lasting way required to say goodbye to limerence permanently, you will need to continue with this subconscious reprogramming for at least three months. At this point, most limerents see evidence that they have effectively replaced their problematic beliefs with and instilled new ones into their mind. They find themselves operating in a completely different way – not only are they entirely over their LO, and incapable of imagining how they once saw them as such a magical, powerful concept, they also emit self-assured, abundant energy and harbour distinct feelings about romance as a facet of life.

Knowing they are more than capable of normal, fulfilling romance that adds flavour to life but does not trigger unsustainable emotional responses, single limerents in this position may be open to opportunities to meet new people and keen to connect with a likeminded partner. Importantly, however, they will feel on a deep, intuitive level that they are simultaneously detached from that potential outcome and in an entirely different headspace to the one they were in before. Their subconscious mind has been rewired; it is no longer motivating them to hunt and *make a beeline for* people to meet their unmet needs, because their needs have been met (Chapter 22) and their beliefs significantly ameliorated. A suitable partner will, for such individuals, be the icing on the cake, not the entire meal itself.

Comparably, most people in a relationship find that they are wholly disinterested in their LO by the three month mark, feeling genuinely immersed in their passions, inspired to connect with their partner and generally stable, safe and content. However, even after you ace the mission of reprogramming your limerence-related beliefs and become immune to the affliction, I highly recommend that you stay committed to **tending to the garden** that is your subconscious mind and seeing *what other favourable changes* you can evoke in your life.

Which beliefs of yours might you be better off shifting? What other, non-romance-related missions seem enticing but out of reach? Whether you have always wanted to generate a stream of passive income, become the fittest version of yourself you could possibly be or even master the art of sleep and get eight consolidated hours a night, the key lies in altering your belief systems. Choose one of the two following techniques (or experiment with both – the goal is just to enter the state that you would be in if you truly believed whatever you want was possible/were experiencing what you want to desire), perform it every night and dare yourself to keep chasing higher and higher calibres of existence once you start seeing results.

1). Self-hypnosis and visualisation:

The premise of this technique is that the brain is very responsive to imagery, whether seen or conjured up by your imagination. While you may not realise it, you are constantly imagining scenes and looping them in your mind. Often, these are negative scenarios that would be unpleasant to experience, such as the detailed depiction of an impending presentation or tricky upcoming conversation going wrong. But, a lot of your imaginal scenes will be positive, productive and already working for you in ways that you are not aware of – ways that you are most likely attributing to outer causes.

The principal goal here is to come up with a mental scene (around 5-15 seconds long) that depicts a scene that would follow you achieving/experiencing what you desire, and then loop it in your head repeatedly until you fall asleep. Some people recommend that you visualise the exciting moment/outcome itself (think: imagining yourself getting married or winning the lottery); however, imaginal movies this emotionally arousing can trigger resistance in beginners. For this reason, I suggest that you instead imagine fairly 'neutral' scenes that would naturally follow your achievement of what you want.

You do not need to see the contents of this scenario as clearly as you would in real life, nor does the scene need to be identical each time you let it run in your mind; this technique is simply a tool **to get you to** *feel* like the person you want to become – to get you to enter a new emotional state. There is also no hard and fast rule regarding how many nights in a row each scene should be looped for, but I recommend conjuring up the same mental imagery every night until you are holding proof of your changed beliefs/mentality **in your hands**.

For example, relating back to limerence, you might realise that three beliefs of yours need to be changed: a). the belief that 'special' people are rare and need to be clung onto, b). the belief that crazy highs and lows are necessary to live a fulfilling life and c). the belief that your LO is the categorically, irrevocably the 'most attractive person in the world'. In this situation, it would be wise to come up with three mental movies that place you in a new reality where i). these beliefs have been replaced with their opposites and ii). you are seeing proof of this around you.

With regards to what to imagine, this comes down to your personal preferences, and what feels most effortless and believable for you; getting The Law of Belief (a newer, more precise term for 'The Law of Assumption') to work for you requires discipline, but no strenuous effort. The subconscious mind is completely **unresponsive to mental coercion**, and wholly responsive to playful, intentionally looped, authentic imagery. You want this process to be light, natural and enjoyable – you want to immerse yourself in your scene like a dreamy child, cutting off your senses so that you are **embodying the version of yourself** that you truly would be were you living it in real life.

When looking to achieve goals that are easily quantifiable, **highly specific scenes** can be an effective way of conveying to your subconscious that you are already the person who naturally achieves such things/that precise thing. This will them stimulate your subconscious mind to a).assimilate new beliefs and b). move you to speak, act, think and feel accordingly. For example, many people opt to imagine scenes featuring them sitting in a circle with their friends and vividly hearing one of them congratulating them on something, signing a large check for their mother, or looking at their Fitbit and seeing that they have surpassed their personal best. If you are in a relationship and limerent, you might want to imagine yourself on holiday with your partner/family feeling completely present, and thinking "thank goodness – how on earth was I ever trapped in limerence?", or "all my psychological needs are met, and I am right <u>where</u> I want to be, <u>with</u> whom I want to be."

Equally, you may find that it feels more genuine, and therefore more momentum-conducive, to simply imagine yourself in a refreshed, abundant mental state, under which lots of **good beliefs are implicit**. There is really no limit to what real-life changes you can achieve through reprogramming your subconscious mind in this more 'diffuse' way as long as **your imaginal scene stirs up emotion**. That is absolutely essential – looping scenes that feel bland, overly-glossy and generic will not communicate what you desire to your subconscious. It does not matter how someone else might gauge *their* success – you need to run mental mini-movies that make *you* enter different, enlivened emotional states and saturate your subconscious mind with the notion of the wish fulfilled, even if these are a little unconventional.

For this reason, many people find it easier to opt for imagery that is slightly more _subtly indicative_ of them having achieved/experienced what they wish to become able to achieve/experience. To help you get over your LO, you could imagine yourself sat at the computer, writing a diary entry or an email to a friend about how you are interested in someone new and have 'realised that your type is actually X (the opposite to your LO's personality)'. Or, you may want to imagine yourself simply **quietly laughing to yourself** about this limerent episode, wondering how/why you ever believed it would be permanent. You can even picture yourself **exactly where you are**, in bed, just 'knowing' that you are now limerence free. If you are in a current relationship, you could imagine yourself joking around with your partner, focusing on them and the nature surrounding you both.

However, short, snappy, laser-focused scenes featuring more conspicuous indications that you are now the person you wish to become will be equally transformative... as long as they make you feel how that version of you would feel, your subconscious mind will, over time, be tricked into believing that you have lived these experiences and, therefore, are now someone who is naturally loved/limerence free/capable of deriving mental stimulation from non-limerent pursuits/financially abundant/a good public speaker/quite literally whatever you want to be.

This is then when the magic happens – as you resume your daily life, you will start to play out this 'character' more and more without even realising. **Bridges of events** will unfold that you don't even notice and things will transpire, until a year later, limerence will be an unrecognisable element of your past. Your mentality, your success and (if you so desire) the people you associate with will be unfathomably different. And the best part? It will all feel so natural that a part of you will wonder whether your subconscious programming has elicited these changes, or whether 'it would have happened anyway'! Hint: it really wouldn't have, had you not had faith in your brain's ability to change and induce different emotions in you, taken action, and grittily pursued the goal of complete subconscious mind reprogramming.

2). Affirmations to Permanently Catapult Yourself Away From Limerence

Now, a small percentage of the population is aphantasic and cannot generate mental imagery at will. Others simply prefer to communicate to their mind in phrases, finding language more of a powerful tool in generating **the right flurry of emotions** (which is, ultimately, the goal of these sessions). I personally vouch for both techniques, and have had marvellous results from combining them both, sometimes even weaving three different scenes and a few affirmations into the same reprogramming session and repeating this for weeks. It would be redundant, at this point in this book, to say that you need to choose affirmations that resonate with you personally and permit *emotional state-shifting*. You will have already grasped the importance of this, for the subconscious mind responds to, and reorganises itself, **in response to emotional experiences**, whether 'naturally triggered' ones or ones that have been intentionally stirred up through imaginal acts.

For some people, biblical or spiritual quotes empower them and allow them to reach **heights of angelic clarity** that regular language doesn't. For many, however, they find the most effective affirmations to be phrases of a more familiar, accessible register that aren't tinged by anything excessively lofty or spiritual. This is completely your choice. Affirmations all, of course, need to be fed to your subconscious mind during the Alpha window before sleep, when your brain is shut off from the world and receptive. However, you can *additionally* mentally rehearse affirmations/think of them during the day. Despite being far less capable of penetrating your subconscious mind while you are wide-awake and engaged with the world (and altering your behaviour/self-concept in a lasting way), they will comfort your conscious mind and **keep you recovery-oriented** and cheerful.

Here are some examples of affirmations that will prove genuinely life-changing to you – in the chapter that you are currently in – if they resonate with you (remember, as you recite or think of them, you want to be feeling **some sort of positive emotion**, even if just a refreshingly calm neutrality/feeling of safety and love that you have not accessed in weeks):

a). Every day, everything is getting better for me *in every way possible*.

b). *Since when have I been* so good at handling my emotions?

c). Evil leaves no mark – I am immune to resentment, pain and jealousy, and avalanches of abundance flow through me constantly.

d). I am constantly riding the wave of good fortune… the odds are always in my favour.

e). Your beliefs are always reflected outwards. By changing my beliefs, I am guaranteed to be automatically lead to the life of my dreams.

f). All of the people in my life are equally special. I have outgrown the illusion that a single person can control my emotions; the truth is always, and has always been, balance, love and light.

g). *Since when* have I been so naturally energetic, positive and free?

h). *I remember when* I once wanted to feel this level of self-fulfilment, childlike enthusiasm, and freedom from illusory psychological afflictions. Finally, I'm free.

i). Anything I turn over to my subconscious mind is expressed. So, subconscious, I intend to be stable, strong and passionate – a lover of life.

You'll notice that some of these affirmations are questions. This is because the subconscious mind loves to problem-solve. Implying that you have already achieved something and, in reflection, are keen to work out why/how you have achieved it is a sly little trick; by prompting your brain to dig around for answers, these affirmation-questions can help to solidify new beliefs remarkably quickly.

Of course, these example affirmations may not resonate with you – you are free to come up with whichever ones you like. They always work if they make you feel how the improved you *would feel,* having received/experienced proof of the beliefs in question being truths. Naturally, a single limerent who has never had a real relationship will have very different beliefs to modify than an affluent businessman/woman who has succeeded in all aspects of their life and has a spouse and children, yet falls into limerence over people they feel 'free' with and 'understood' by. I trust that you will be able to craft **exquisite affirmations** that are perfect for *your* circumstances and current belief systems.

Trust Your Subconscious Mind and Watch the Magic Pan Out

While employing these regimens, you must forget about the 'how'; the language of the subconscious mind is <u>emotion and playfulness,</u> not pragmatic, ego-driven, strategic planning. You do not need to ascertain how future partners treating you with respect is actually going to pan out in full detail, or, if you are married, which precise conversations you may end up having with your spouse once you are limerence-free. Or which of *their* personality traits you are going to start to admire once again.

If imagining these hypothetical scenarios feels pleasantly emotionally evocative to you and generates feelings that are in consonance with you believing that you are in your **new, ameliorated reality,** then by all means incorporate them into your visualisation/affirmation sessions. But, if they are stressful or leave you feeling like there are too many possibilities – too many undetermined factors – and that changing your beliefs and eventually holding this new life in your hands is 'going to be hard work', ignore them. Your subconscious is immensely powerful, constantly running to move you towards goals and outcomes. You can relax into the knowing that it will elicit exactly the right behaviour/responses/actions from you in the right moments to get you what you want to be and to align you with who you want. As long as you take charge and <u>command it to focus</u> on the outcomes that you truly desire, from the position of already having reached them.

Speaking to Your Subconscious Mind Alters the Wirings of Your Deep, <u>Unconscious Brain</u>

The unconscious brain constantly orchestrates a plethora of physiological processes deep in your viscera (internal organs) to perfectly match the homeostatic requirements of your body before it enters a negative energy balance. This anticipatory monitoring is referred to as **allostasis**, and is carried out extremely efficiently around the clock. It is possible because the brain receives constant input from the entire body (a process called **interoception**). *Everything* from a). tactile sensations, like someone brushing against you, b). visceral input, such as a generous load of buttered cabbage being deposited into your stomach, and c). the temporal pattern of visual stimuli associated with you expectedly spotting your friend in a gaudy fluorescent green anorak is communicated to the brain. Some of this is brought into your consciousness, enabling you to realise that you are staring at your friend, rather than a stranger, or that, despite fancying a slice of chocolate cake, you are actually full to the brim with cruciferous vegetables and are better off politely saying no.

We remain unconscious, however, to most of the stimuli that we are bombarded with – this is absolutely essential to our growth, survival and reproductive fitness of our species. If you were constantly aware of everything you were digesting, your blood pressure down to every fine fluctuation and your bile secretion status, you would be intellectually and practically hindered. Fascinatingly, we are also unaware of much that goes on within our own brain – we normally cannot decipher why we are suddenly feeling peppier than usual, why we are crying and ruminating over our LO despite thinking we were getting better, and why the whiff of lavender we have just received has transported us back to a memory of being in school.

We may *think* we can intuit our own psychology well, but we can only really run predictions and go off past patterns; the true workings of our unconscious brains remain hidden to us. What is certain, however, is that the brain is always ticking and determining our a). physiological status and b). psychological status. I have illustrated this point with rudimentary examples, but all of your mental modalities, from your emotional 'set-point' (the baseline feeling you tend to return to), your daily energy levels and your interest or disinterest in opportunities that come your way during the work day are all finely controlled by brain centres that work behind the scenes. In other words, this information is not brought to your awareness.

The way to communicate with these brain regions and ultimately alter their modes of action is **through the subconscious mind**, which is most accessible and ready to mould itself to your commands during states of wakeful relaxation.

The Law of Belief Mysteriously, But Undeniably, Governs All

I cannot stress this enough – whether you are a student, retired, single, married with children or in a complex polyamorous relationship, your beliefs are ultimately what will determine whether your limerent mentality is channelled as a). actual, debilitating limerence, or b). passion, productivity and joy in all other areas of your life. In accord with this, there is no single facet of your life that is not mappable to very precise beliefs that you unknowingly hold to be true. Some of these hunches will, of course, be 'true' in line with the rules of consensus reality, e.g. 'reliable people aren't normally late to meetings', and 'I feel better and radiate more enthusiasm when I exercise regularly. These are fine, and can be left unperturbed – allowing them to direct you on autopilot is unlikely to hold you back from achieving your goals and living a life that is rewarding for you. A lot of ideas you 'intuit' to be inarguably true, however, particularly the negative ones, will be warped, compromising, inaccurate conclusions about real life that are either getting in your way or sabotaging you entirely, depending on their severity. You must start to consider addressing and supplanting these as important as you would deem studying for an exam that you desired a good grade in, or putting in hours of strength-training to grow more lean muscle mass.

The implications of all of this can, of course, be wrapped up as follows: what is best for you – mentally stimulating, aesthetically pleasing, the right level of comforting - will only be brought into your experience if you stay faithful to watching your mental diet and *continually* overriding any beliefs that are in discord with the idea that these things are feasible and achievable for you. The same applies to successfully transitioning through the limerence recovery process and emerging immune to the state. Now that you realise the power of your subconscious and its ability to be tamed, you should only encourage the momentum of thoughts, beliefs, notions, assumptions and predictions that you want to see grow and be expressed outwards.

29. Limerent Objects and the Fantasy Bond

Now that we have expounded how to practically recover from limerence in depth, it is about time that we address the fact that it takes two to tango. You are genetically and, currently, psychologically vulnerable to limerence, but to engage your reward system vigorously enough to create true person addiction and a fantasy bond, someone must a). intermittently reward you and b). possess traits that result in them generating feelings in you that counteract your internalised pain and suffering.

As can be deduced from talking to anyone who has experienced limerence, LOs are nearly always emotionally-disordered and chaotic to a certain extent. Only unusual, noncommittal people with personality disorders a). will radiate energy uncontrolled and raw enough to soothe whatever wounding you have (when a securer partner will not flood you with this *intensity*) and b). will not run a mile when they realise that *you* are besotted by them and *they* are looking for a relationship. We are not talking about typical unrequited love or crushes, here – we are talking about a severe state of psychiatric imbalance that harrowingly warps your reality while you succumb to it. Only people who are, themselves, dealing with unmet needs and/or are unusually narcissistic are going to keep you on their radar when you are notably suffering and in a compromised psychological state triggered by *them*.

Limerent feelings very rarely go unnoticed; your energy towards your LO will most likely betray you, regardless of how composed you try to act with them (or normally are). Furthermore, normal adults will be repelled to some degree (although hopefully act compassionately, of course) upon discovering that someone adores them with reckless abandon when they do not share those dreamy feelings. However, LOs typically do not speak up and address the elephant in the room, namely your state of **unrequited lovesickness**. Why is this? It may be that your LO is genuinely oblivious to your feelings, due to your connection being fantastical (i.e. non-existent) or their possessing abnormal empathy deficits. However, it is just as likely that they shy away from addressing the obvious because something about your unusual connection <u>makes them feel good</u>. When you exude unconstrained admiration and awe, you are helping them deal with their own shortcomings and pain by affirming to them that they are loved/attractive/powerful/special/relevant (*whatever* it is that they want to feel).

Your **trigger archetype** for LOs may be narcissists in positions of authority who start to flirt and engage with you before pulling back, or they could be easily excitable, frivolous and carefree souls who start to show the stereotypic array of borderline personality disorder (BPD) traits after initially enmeshing with you. As it is curated by psychological factors that are unique to you and based on your genetics and life experience, ascertaining what archetype of person attracts you in this wild way is immensely revealing. You may fall for a LO who is relatively normal but intermittently rewards you *just enough* to tap into that idealised concept of **a detached 'saviour'** that you have in your head. The next one, however, may seem more potent to you from the beginning, display some toxic traits, fascinate you with their ability to treat life like a game and ultimately leave you all alone and in the deepest state of limerence known to man.

Considering a). what all of your past LOs have had in common and b). how both the ecstasy and the lows triggered in you by these people has varied will let you into the secret buried deep in your subconscious mind: that you need to create a different life for yourself that fulfils you and to kiss goodbye to unrequited, impossible love as a coping mechanism.

30. The Dangers of Analysing Your Limerent Object's Behaviour

I consciously chose not to start this book with an in-depth analysis of the character traits that LOs normally have, because doing so would perpetuate the myth that it is *their* fault that we become limerent. This is not a moral stance of mine, as many LOs are indeed nasty and deserving of a wake-up call that may shift them towards taking some responsibility for how they treat others. Rather, I have avoided centring this book around the unbridled analysis of toxic personality types because there is a difference between what is interesting and what is *relevant to recovery*. Limerence awakens a profound interest in psychology and the nuances of the human mind in all sufferers; in addition to being the epitome of the brain submitting us to unnecessary pain, it additionally demonstrating how interpersonal relationships can edge into the realm of the surreal, absurd and downright damaging. Few phenomena on this earth are more fascinating if you are analytical but also emotionally-intelligent and intrigued by people.

However, there is a difference between a). seeing your own limerence issue as a puzzle to crack away at and overcome and b). hyper-focusing on the **actions of your past LOs/current LO** to the point of self-sabotage. Refrain from erroneously believing that your freedom from limerence lies in meticulously analysing how you have been treated by these people, developing a sense of indignant anger at what you have endured and committing to writing off similar individuals in the future. Entertaining this attitude will keep you addicted to the person you have in mind, as the opposite of love is not hate, but indifference. Allowing yourself to get worked up about this person and fixating on them/their own psychological issues for months is synonymous to trapping yourself in a recovery 'farce': convinced that you're moving forward, but still caught up in the depths of person addiction.

Even if someone bonds with you intensely and then detaches, leaving you heartbroken, growing vindictive towards cluster B personality disorders traits and 'promising to never let yourself fall for narcissists again' *alone* will not render you immune to them. Of course, you must elucidate which traits in your LO evoked such interest in you so that you can carry out the relevant self-work, but this is as far as this mission should go while you are vulnerable. Remember, recovering from a behavioural addiction as notoriously stubborn as limerence involves <u>the absolute renouncement</u> of a life **with limerence at its centre**. There is no real difference between engaging in online Reddit discussions about all that your LO has done wrong and stalking their social media obsessively on your own. To your brain, these actions further confirm your LO's status as a complex, omnipotent mass of energy who can dictate your mood at the click of its fingers. Intuitively, it will also interpret this line of focus as you <u>choosing to stay floating down the limerent river</u>, and water will gush along accordingly. When there are so many different bodies of water to dip into, why not climb out of this limiting one that submits you to pain and false hope?

I will reaffirm that pondering which personality disorder may best describe your LOs and reminiscing in full on why you initially felt so drawn to them is essential; doing so will let you in on which **psychological factors of yours** need to be transformed, so that you can become immune to these people. Realise that they are narcissistic, textbook cases of BPD, histrionic or simply *well-meaning but lacking boundaries*, deduce what you need to think and feel to stop matching their frequency, and pull yourself up to emotional freedom. This is a highly constructive (and essential) way to evaluate limerence and find the answers you seek, while false recovery, in contrast, only shifts your focus to your LO even more and perpetuates the heady allure of the addiction. The latter is a dead-end, albeit one that, just like fantasising about a future with your LO, will reward you with dopamine because it will be falsely perceived by your brain as <u>anticipation of more of your LO's affection</u>.

If affairs of the human mind fascinate you, welcome to the club – by all means, immerse yourself in neuroscience and psychology to better understand yourself and others; this is something I actively recommend. Let the revelations that you are having about relationships, authenticity and humanity as a whole stay with you and empower you. However, question the intentions of your subcortical, 'emotional' brain. Do not let it fool you into believing that **bubbling with rage towards your LO** or committing to analysing the factors that may have led to them embodying a particular personality archetype can ever be conducive to recovery. This flips the focus of your pathological person addiction without changing its intensity or treating it; whether you are idealising their illusory god-like qualities or writing diary entries about their nuanced and complex mind, you are still focusing on them as an enormous, blazing, powerful entity capable of dictating your mood. You must instead focus on becoming a superior version of *yourself*, so that this very illusion can be shattered and the boundaries separating them from <u>the realm of other mortal, normal humans</u> dissolved.

31. The Role That Intermittent Reinforcement Plays in Limerence

LOs cannot be discussed without us touching on intermittent reward schedules, for their flighty, erratic behaviour and hot-and-cold moods do nothing but intermittently reinforce limerents. Your genetics and experience render you prone to falling for a specific type of person (your trigger archetype), but at the end of the day, the dopaminergic reward pathways are impartial to how this person looks, talks or acts. Whether you are drawn to steel-cold narcissistic personality disorder (NPD) individuals or histrionic, dramatic whirlwinds who are, themselves, needy, limerence involves you being sporadically rewarded with their attention and yearning for more.

If LOs were not somewhat unpredictable, it would be virtually impossible for you to pass from the initial glimmer into complete neurochemical addiction and dependence. Some research carried out in the 1950s by behaviourist Skinner does a great job at illustrating how we mammals fall hard for rewards that are not offered consistently. Concerning operant conditioning, this work of his involved placing mice in a simple operant conditioning chamber (a.k.a. a Skinner box) and training them to press a lever to receive an edible reward. Initially, continuous reinforcement was applied; the mice received food whenever they successfully pressed the lever. Once they learnt to associate the lever-pressing with the release of food (and this manipulation of the dispenser became firmly integrated into their *behavioural repertoire*), they were submitted to **variable-interval schedules**. For example, they would press the lever twice and receive two pellets as they expected, but then would not receive any more for sixty seconds. After this whole minute of ceaseless attempts despite zero responsiveness from the feeding unit, they would see three bites of food appear at once and delightedly chomp them down.

This intermittent reinforcement schedule worked frighteningly well in pushing these mice right into the clutches of addiction. Instead of growing frustrated and deciding to stop engaging in the pursuit of the reward when the **reward contingencies** became unpredictable, the mice started to push the lever more frantically and hung around the feeding area like moths hugging a bright lamp. Skinner described this behaviour as 'hard to extinguish', and all mammals respond similarly to rewards that are intermittently provided. We start to become consumed by the possibility of getting the reward soon, and fretful and dysphoric when it seems to not be arriving. Consider gambling or betting – just like how not everyone is prone to limerence, not everyone can be readily lured in by an addiction of this nature, but we *are* all more motivated to play with money when we do not know when we will get lucky.

NB: studies reveal that mice and humans alike are not nearly as captured by the unpredictable sprinkling of food, affection or drugs when it is very rare and hardly given from the beginning. What really carves out deep, desperate addiction is when they are **initially rewarded enough** for their brain to learn when to expect the reward and *then* submitted to more sporadic treatment. Often the most agonising limerences occur when a real phase of bonding did occur between you and your LO before they cut the relationship short, even if this was just you two chatting as classmates.

However, of course, other limerents somehow latch onto LOs who have barely spoken to them. This occurs because their imagination takes off when they first start to notice this person (they are still hopeful, imagining various outcomes and oblivious that they will never live out these dreams in real life). The result is that the brain believes that they *have really experienced* consistent, predictable doses of this person's attention. When they start to see just how unrequited their love is, they wake up to how intermittent and meaningless a lot of these corridor smiles, Facebook likes and drunken phone calls really are. Therefore, from your brain's perspective (being easily tricked), **all manifestations of limerence** can be considered to involve 'reliable signs of interest followed by intermittent signs of interest'. Even if you never truly bonded with your LO, your brain thinks you did, and you're now addicted because their energy/personality complements your unmet needs in an unusual way. Connecting with them (whether in a real or partially imagined way) felt good, and you want more.

So, we know that those who experience limerence are extremely receptive to intermittent reinforcement; the two go hand in hand. Depending on your relationship with your LO, they will be intermittently rewarding you in different ways, despite the underlying neural mechanisms being identical. If you are limerent over one of your closest friends, maybe they occasionally look at you with a certain intensity that makes you wonder whether they truly consider the connection platonic. Just as you start to analyse 'what you are', however, they transition back to joking around they view you as a sibling… until you two meet for a drink a month later and the bond seems to take on a romantic tone again. This abstract, perplexing type of social dance ("will we, won't we?") is very common in limerence; LOs are unpredictable people who are *unable* to relate to us normally, and we are prone to latching on and deifying them. Two wrongs certainly do not make a right – the result is a strange, boundaryless relationship between two people. You fall obsessively in love to your detriment, while your LO (normally) skips around you, happy to stay connected despite your true feelings being quite obvious.

However, of course, the extent to which your LO's behaviour is 'questionable/immature/unpredictable' depends on *your* **unmet needs, beliefs and self-concept** (i.e. what it takes to get *you* to see the glimmer in someone and fall into full-blown limerence). It may be that your LO is not someone you have *ever even* had a real conversation with, let alone someone who sometimes shows partial romantic interest in you and 'strings you along'. If this is the case, and you feel silly and as if your case of limerence is 'more delusional' than most, do not beat yourself up; regular communication and a real bond with the object of your affection is not a prerequisite to being affected by intermittent reward, as we have touched on above. If they are a mere acquaintance who you find physically, mentally and spiritually attractive and they occasionally like your Facebook posts, that can very well submit you to highs and lows that are *just as strong* as our other examples that involve more substantial exchanges. In extreme cases, limerents **fall for celebrities** they've never met, further proving just how illusory and ill-founded the romantic feelings that this condition elicits can be.

After all, the brain has evolved to work in a way that latches us onto things that enhance our mood, aid us in food location and let us survive long enough to pass on our genetic material, and it often gets things very wrong. The more primitive modes of action of your brain are absolutely nothing to be ashamed of, nor can you control them *before you learn* that you are manifesting limerence by allowing them to chronically spiral in the first place. For that reason, I respond to everyone who reaches out to me with the same unconditional compassion. Their LO may be someone who they have dated in real life or someone they have merely smiled at a few times in the office, but I do not care – if someone tells me that they are in mental agony, I wholly believe them because I am a neuroscientist. The human brain is capable of many miraculous things, and a side effect of this is that we occasionally endure life chapters of horrific mental health in response to no real dangers. Pain is pain, and I am here to help as many limerents transform their subconscious minds as I can without judging them in the slightest.

But, becoming (and staying) so smitten with someone you've never properly spoken to may indicate that you have **more self-work to do** than someone who, for example, is hung up in this way over an ex-partner. I say this because a *particularly* heightened degree of delusionality does accompany such cases of limerence that involve a lack of a 'real connection' with your LO. Even if you consciously know that your chances of dating in real life are tiny, your brain is nonetheless conjuring up a potently strong illusion from a complete absence of *real life information*. This doesn't mean you're crazy – the mere fact that you can contemplate that you might be fortunately reveals that you are not. However, the fact that your brain's able to subject you to such horrible emotional lows in response to the realisation that you two are not, in actual fact, together, does reveal that you have <u>very severe unmet needs</u>.

This individual's **mere 'imaginary presence'** in your life (whether they're a distant acquaintance you've never spoken to but later searched online, or a famous artist who's deep lyrics speak to you on a different level) is capable of eliciting such intense emotions in you because your brain <u>believes that you desperately need them</u>. After all, if you were in dire need of a particular type of medication, you'd certainly be responsive to images of it on the Internet; the same goes for primitive needs like hunger and thirst – if you are **ravenous or parched**, the sound of food or drink being served can instantly assuage tension, fear and even make you feel pre-emptively replenished. But, we simply should not, and cannot, allow our responses to people to be so markedly reactive in adulthood. Of course, the way to solve this issue (and stop it ever arising again) is to become a version of yourself that is *not desperate for them* in the first place. This is, after all, the premise of all of the techniques that have so far been presented in this book.

32. The Benefits of the Limerent Disposition

Those of you capable of experiencing true, scarlet-red, shatteringly painful limerence are blessed and cursed. The same disposition that renders you higher up the spectrum for diagnosable conditions like OCD and primes you for love addiction also confers you with many unique, idiosyncratic perks. This **duality** to the neural basis of limerence is quite fascinating, and is rarely talked about; after all, limerents seek high-quality material to educate themselves and recover as quickly as possible. The side effect of this can be a tendency to shun and hide away the fact that you are limerence-prone.

What this strategy overlooks, however, is the fact that we can never alter our genetics and change our fundamental nature. Of course, by attacking the root psychological causes of limerence, we can outgrow the condition, leave behind LOs and launch ourselves into a dreamlike existence – this is exactly what I want you to do when you finish reading this book. However, I do not want you to try and suppress your perfectionistic, obsessive nature entirely, nor your ability to immerse yourself in abstract concepts, your interest in other people, your emotional intelligence or your creativity. These are all examples of traits that accompany the ability to become limerent, which can, similarly, be traced back to the neurotransmission that we covered in the first section of this book. The last thing that I want you to do is to think that you need to become someone more 'conventional', emotionally-flat and unreactive, because this is a). impossible (suppression never equals healing) and, importantly, b). entirely unnecessary.

Serial limerents are normally quick-witted, verbally-expressive, perceptive, emotionally-astute, analytical lovers of life; I am yet to help someone suffering from limerence who has not had a beautiful command of their first language (if not several), some unusual hobbies and a great degree of interest in affairs of the human mind. This curious essence does not need to be tampered with in any way, and this is why I treat limerence in the way that I do; the wonderful thing about considering the pathology from a psychological-verging-on-spiritual perspective is that it allows you to spot-treat your psyche, *only* altering elements that do not serve you.

At the end of the day, limerence is an organic, primitive response to love that you need to pull yourself out of – an aberrant, pathological experience of romance. Taking an anti-depressant will do nothing but temporarily dull your pain (in addition to submitting you to a whole host of other side effects). But, meeting your needs ruthlessly and determinedly and stepping up and controlling your belief systems rewires your brain and promotes neural healing *naturally*… without you meddling with your neurons' firing by inhibiting serotonin uptake (and dealing with unpleasant off-target effects). In other words, a). employing all of the psychological techniques described in this book and b). assimilating, and remembering, what limerence truly is (i.e. staying as impartial as possible/rejecting delusional thoughts) is ALSO going to treat you at the **neuroscientific/neural level**.

So, beating limerence (or any mental condition) is not a matter of choosing between neuroscience and 'softer' psychology/spirituality. The superior techniques will always seem more 'holistic', but will actually be working their magic behind the scenes at the molecular/neural level, too. Altering your belief systems, constructing a new sense of self and meeting your unmet needs profoundly and beneficially alters your brain, because **your psychology is never dissociable** from its biological underpinnings.

Any technique that leaves you feeling happier, stronger and freer, whether it's subconscious mind reprogramming for limerence or exposure therapy for a phobia, is actually promoting neural rewiring and remedying your neurotransmitter imbalances better (and more precisely!) than any psychiatric drug ever could. That's not to say that they aren't ever useful – certain conditions like psychosis are best managed with medication. However, minimal potential lies in their ability to effectively treat behavioural patterns like limerence – a low dose of an antidepressant may take the edge off rumination/pain without inducing profound 'dulling' effects in responsive individuals, but they will always be prone to falling for future LOs the second that they come off the drug. Unless you do the work required to **immunise yourself against all LOs** (and limerence itself), you are merely balancing a plaster over the problem.

If you treat the overarching psychological root causes of limerence, on the other hand, you are guaranteed to leave the condition behind and surface as a new, more resilient, cheerful version of yourself. What's more, you will not lose your ability to engage in tasks in an obsessive way or research things on the Internet for hours, your tendency to experience rich, interesting emotions or your general zeal for life.

Importantly, challenging this energy into something *other* than person addiction will give you an edge over many other people you know, who follow the herd, never feel intense, unbridled emotions and who are incapable of seeing life as an expansive simulation in which it is possible to achieve our dreams. To serve as an example, I do not think I would have the drive or the incentive to write lots of online material and this book while also working as a neuroscientist if I did not possess the genes that *used to* let me be limerent and miserable.

Despite being unable to relate to people who are disinterested in engaging their brains obsessively, I have benefitted from my limerent mentality more than I could ever convey using human language. I spent my childhood immersed in books, hobbies and was always innovating and creating; my parents used to tell me that 'when I decided to do something, that thing was mine and no one could beat me'. While proud parental commentary must be taken with a grain of salt (!), it is certainly true that I have always had an incredibly strong, manic passion for (and commitment) to the things that I love. To stay limerence-immune, I, personally, must constantly endeavour to quench my insatiable desire for intensity, spontaneity and authenticity – to connect with new, quirky people with interesting life missions, and to hear their stories. To let myself be saturated by their energy, albeit in a healthy, sustainable way. Being able to pursue things and projects that allow me to unleash my goal-oriented focus is also of the utmost importance to me. In order to meet these crucial needs of mine, I ensure that I never grow complacent. I consider every day an opportunity to edge a little closer towards mastery of a new language, the completion of a project (like this book) or any other meaningful goal that resonates with me and **unlocks emotions** in me that I enjoy.

While things got dark once I hit the age of fourteen and started experiencing horrific, dizzying limerent pain that I did not have the tools or the knowledge to deal with, I still excelled in my studies and always had a clear idea that I wanted to take neuroscience as far as I could take it. Psychology, foreign languages, animals and writing also set my soul on fire. You see, being limerence-prone allows you to *generally* experience non-tangible things in an intense way; if you are genetically-prone, you have an impressive imagination that can contemplate abstract things and weave up convincing narratives very quickly. And, influenced by these narratives, your subconscious mind will automatically send you down a path towards whatever actions it believes will make these things **externalise in your reality**.

While you are currently experiencing this mental driving force in an unwanted, bothersome way, you must allow the true extent of your potential to dawn on you. You have been born equipped with the **ideal neural machinery for manifestation**. Instead of letting your mind be inundated by illusory conversations with your LO or the fantasy of you two getting married, focus on other concepts that excite and scare you, such as moving to a new country within the next two years, reconnecting with all of your childhood friends, connecting with a new social group that makes you feel 'different', starting a small business or embarking on a fitness journey.

33. Discipline the Flame, But Do Not Stifle It

Limerence involves mania, depression, regret and intense existentialism. However, I like to consider our unruly limerent energy as a golden, glowing mass that can be directed towards other areas in our lives to produce astonishing things. The presence of this duality is, of course, not unique to limerence; anorexia nervosa is a great example of a tenacious condition underpinned by a mentality that, if overcome, actually gives sufferers an immense step up in life. The neuroticism and perfectionism of ritualised starvation reflect a very keen sense of motivation and a strong affinity for goal-oriented thinking. Typically very academically-gifted as children, post-recovery anorexics often start businesses, excel in their careers and master niche skills.

Just like a limerent in the crystallisation phase of the disorder, when ill, anorexic individuals are not tapping into their true essence; they are starving themselves in order to feel better about whatever it is in their life that they wish to control but (falsely) believe that **they cannot control**. Redirecting their focus away from systemisation of food and an obsession with calories and towards something else allows them to live a life that they never dreamed they could have while trapped by their addiction to dieting. Interestingly, limerence involves a similar **proclivity for goal-oriented behaviour**; after all, no one sets and maintains a goal quite like a limerent believing that it will edge him or her closer to his/her LO. Whether that means losing a significant amount of weight to look svelte in an outfit at a party that their LO may attend six months down the line, or reading four enormous books that their LO has listed as their favourites in a social media post, they will be fuelled on by dopamine and adrenaline and will succeed.

Give yourself your best chance and unleash this whirlwind focus onto other aspects of your life, but ensure to pick goals that both truly thrill *and* scare you, just as limerence does. Plan that podcast, write that poetry book or quit your job and start that eCommerce business. You will reap so many rewards that you will look back and no longer resent being limerence-susceptible - the upsides to expressing this phenotype are frankly splendid. Simultaneously, you will, of course, need to ensure you are learning to meet your psychological needs as well as you possibly can and, being at the absolute crux of limerence recovery, religiously implement the **subconscious reprogramming strategies** we discussed in depth in Chapter 28.

You can consider fostering the growth of new, exciting beliefs, transforming your mentality and becoming permanently immune to limerence like constructing a **complex, robust automated system**. Despite taking time and effort to establish, it will permanently yield wonderful results once set into motion, occasionally requiring some maintenance touches but never again needing to be built from scratch.

Your subconscious mind is always influencing your emotional and physiological health, and learning to command it will render you magnetic to avalanches of success in all aspects of your life – that I do not say lightly. Suspend your disbelief and commit to recovering from limerence, even if it is all you have known. Nothing in life is easy, nor should it be. However, visions of a better future that are backed by faith and paired with the drive to succeed are guaranteed to unfold.

34. Real Stories From Real Limerents

This chapter was not present in the first edition of *The Limerent Mind*. I have since come back to add it in because I believe that it is just what you need. Here, we have six poignant, evocative, lively accounts from six real limerents in different stages of recovery. Names (and a few details) have been changed as per their requests, but the essences of all of these individuals' stories remain untouched.

Being a collection of (somewhat) short stories, you are free to read them as you please – to devour them all at once, enjoy them one-by-one, or put this final section aside until you gain traction in your own recovery and feel like immersing yourself in them. I am confident that the range of feelings, themes, experiences and LO dynamics that they convey will prove invaluable in helping you piece together everything that you have learnt from this book. That you will be able to draw strong parallels between their stories and your own. And that you will find doing so fascinating, enriching and, at times, amusing. Because, at the end of the day, limerence is a human state, and one that we must learn to laugh at a little.

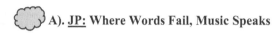 **A). <u>JP:</u> Where Words Fail, Music Speaks**

I'm writing to you in response to your call for limerents' stories on your website.

Firstly I want to thank you for your involvement in dissecting and clarifying this 'disease' that haunts so many of us. Reading your articles helped me a lot after I first went no contact (NC) – it is obvious that you speak the limerent 'language', and I felt understood because of this.

I am a divorced guy in his early fifties, living a pretty boring and lonely life, with few friends and contacts beside work and family. I had been working alone from home for several months when I became **limerent for a celebrity musician half my age**. This is a first for me – in the past I only really fell limerent for people I knew personally, and who were in my age range.

I've decided to send you my story, even if it's rather boring, in the hope of raising awareness about **celebrity limerence**. I guess that I also wrote it out as an excuse to think about my LO once again… while in NC.

I've frequented celebrity obsession forums and limerence forums, without feeling at home in any of them. I'm pretty sure I was mostly seen as having *imaginary problems* by posters on those specifically about limerence – many of them were going truly insane, and fighting to keep their family and friends. A lot of people on the celebrity obsession forums seemed to have serial, life-long issues with falling for people they had never met. Weirdly enough, they seemed to partly enjoy their obsessions, which was something I did not relate to at all.

For me this limerent episode (LE) has really just felt like my past LEs, with the difference being that my LO is somebody I've never met face to face, and the disadvantage being that I have had a lot more 'sources' to feed my limerence. As an atheist, the onset of this current LE was **the closest thing to magic** I've ever experienced. It was so unexpected, intense and irrational that I suddenly understood why men used to accuse women of witchcraft in the Dark Ages.

I first saw my LO on a recommended YouTube video, about 11 months ago, and didn't even like her music initially. However, her on-stage persona – an **unconventional, fairylike girl**… albeit kind, authentic, and full of passion – instantly captured my attention and made me want to know more about her. So I started to watch her interviews and music videos. Over the course of the subsequent two weeks, I slowly fell in love with her voice and music. Naïve and innocent, **I searched the web for 'music addiction'** and similar topics, seeking to understand why I could not stop listening to her music.

After two weeks passed, I realised that, although it was totally irrational and unbelievable, I was actually **starting to feel in love** with this musician… even if there was a huge age gap and I didn't really know her, but rather, a projected image of her. But that image of her – a funny, weird, emphatic, down to earth and authentic girl, with a voice out of this world – was **magnetic to me beyond my understanding**. To be honest, back then, I thought that falling in love with celebrities only happened to lunatic stalkers who ended up in the news. I've never known anyone in real life with this 'problem'. I, myself, had never even been a fan of a celebrity before, nor interested in any celebrities' lives – let alone fallen in love with one.

At that point, remembering my past painful LEs for real life people, I started to fear the worst and tried to cut myself off from her, going cold turkey. I guess I was also trying to show myself that I'm not one of those lunatic stalkers who makes the news. Despite this 'cut off', she still was in my mind every minute. Detaching from my feelings felt awful, like I was willingly and stupidly **renouncing my one chance of heaven**. I only made it to the day five mark, and then let myself go completely. I listened to her music for hours each day, watched her interviews, and scoured the Internet for information/pictures of her and so on.

This pretence of 'trying to get over her' went on for months. After a while, driven by the immense amount of pain that the addiction was causing me (*sometimes I even had stomach cramps* remembering her voice singing a specific song), I started to limit my listening sessions to 'only' about 10 hours weekly, and also tried to limit the online content centred on her that I was consuming. **I tried to be a mere fan** by joining a fan forum, a first and colossal step for me as I've always detested social media. I also tried to keep my daydreaming about meeting and talking to her *in check*. I managed to create a resemblance of 'normality' for myself– discussing regular things about her with other 'regular fans' helped me in this sense. What I never really managed, however, was to **control the crazy 'discussions' I was having with her in my head**. Whenever I did anything during the day, I felt like I was 'explaining' it to her or something – like she was always there, sharing my every waking moment with me.

I was always in ecstasy while I listened to her music rollerblading, dreaming about her... only to come home and stumble across some info reminding me of all of the reasons why we'd never be together. Then, I'd fall in the *deepest despair and agony*. It was like I actually had two addictions, one for her voice and music, and another one for her... clearly, these two addictions were fuelling each other. I felt a constant tension in me, felt that something was missing... that something wasn't right. That I should do something about it. Apparently, **she was single and alone a lot** because of the COVID restrictions, was fuelling my daydreams about meeting her and, by some miracle, ending up living together, happily. At least for a while.

There's something I must clarify, here. *Rationally*, I knew that no sane girl in her mid-twenties would be attracted to a fifty-year-old guy, let alone a celebrity with a tonne of options. But, a part of me clung onto hope. After all, she was quite far from a normal girl, and I'm pretty far from a normal guy, so who knows – what if she saw *something special* in me? The 'what if' kept me hooked, kept me clinging onto a crazy sliver of optimism. But, I'd simultaneously remind myself that I was losing my mind – that even if we did end up together, I'd probably eventually become bored, anyway. This is precisely what happened with my last LO (**I actually married her, only to divorce from her**). At my age, I am, of course, more than aware that these big loves can die. And if they don't die, that they morph into something calmer. That expecting anything else is delusional – that love, therefore, should never be your sole focus in life.

I feel like there's something I should add: for some reason **I've never had sexual dreams about her**, but then again, I was never intensely sexually attracted to any of my past real-life LOs - maybe with the exception of the previous one, who I dated. Also, bizarrely, I didn't even find this girl **sublimely beautiful** – in some pictures of hers, I actually found her outright ugly. To be honest, if I saw her walking down the street and didn't know who she was, I would probably not even give her a second look. It was her aura, her talents and her emotional depth that really sparkled to me and got me hooked.

I'll admit, I did some very weird things during this period of my LE. Like spending days reading about the music industry, in an attempt to estimate her income. In the end, I found out that this is public information in her country. I was somehow relieved to discover that our net incomes were at least of the same order of magnitude (she is not a hugely well-known musician).

At one point, I actually planned to go on holiday to her hometown **for the slim chance of randomly encountering her in the streets** – the quarantine imposed by her country saved me from this stunt, luckily! I also nearly bought the identical model of piano that she had in her room, despite having never played the instrument in my life. **I started to learn her native language**, only to abandon it because I didn't like it, even if it sounds dreamy when she speaks it. Occasionally, I'd feel something eerily 'switch' in me, as if I was suddenly seeing the world through her eyes, or that she was looking through mine. One day, I even dug around online to assess the chance I had of *breathing a particle of air expired by her* in her hometown, thousands of kilometres away... it felt like magic, and madness. Complete and utter madness.

I was working from home all this time, and my performance was severely affected. For months, I severely struggled to focus on my work, and was actually amazed that nobody commented on my greatly reduced efficiency. My work ethic and attitude was just plummeting.

Acting under the premise of being an innocent, earnest fan, I decided to find out where she lived – her exact address. I knew she actively tried to keep her home address hidden; during live streams that she'd record from her home, she'd even mention that she's a little paranoid by nature. That she doesn't want us, her fans, to find out exactly where she lives. I took this as a sort of challenge and, using small pieces of information already available online, **managed to locate her home address**.

After celebrating my cyber detective skills, I was immediately bombarded by mental imagery. Lots of **real life stalking plans haunted me**, nonstop. She lives in another country and it was impossible for me to actually go there, because of the COVID situation, but this didn't stop me from planning future ways to meet her 'by chance' in her hometown, or from thinking about what mail I could send to her home address. Sometimes, I'd even think about how I'll probably be dead in thirty years. Shouldn't I at least try to get close to the only person who makes me feel alive? Other times, I'd worry about my mental sanity and wonder if I should seek professional help. I even **studied the stalking laws in her country**.

During this daydreaming frenzy, a video of her doing a small dance was posted online. She had filmed it herself, during a work break at the music studio, late at night and in the presence of a band colleague. I suddenly felt the sharp teeth of jealousy cutting deep into me – *she looked so joyful*, while I felt miserable. And **what were they doing there so late?!** After spending a little while in agony, I had a moment of clarity, horrified that I was actually upset that a stranger was having a *small happy moment* during her work break. I felt both sick with jealousy and appalled at my childishness. At the end of the day, I suddenly thought "**** this!", and started to furiously delete all of the bookmarks, pictures and music that I'd been storing on my computer. That anger and disgust at myself helped me to commit to NC seriously, for the first time.

I've now been in NC for about two months, and it's during this period that **I've found out about limerence** for the first time in my life. Previously, I thought that it was simply *my way of falling in love* – with a crazy intensity, involving painful, year-long obsessions. Of course, my NC has not been without the odd relapse. For example, two weeks in, I stumbled by chance upon a picture of her on the Internet and made the mistake of looking at it for a few seconds – probably just five seconds. My heartrate instantly doubled and a rush of adrenaline washed over me. Right afterwards, I once again felt that familiar pain – that knowing that I'll never be with her – and it lasted a whole day. One day of suffering for five seconds of joy. One other time, I was a little drunk and visited the fan forum again. Luckily, my tired state rendered that visit less impactful on me.

After two weeks of NC, I was delighted to notice that sometimes fifteen minutes passed without her even crossing my mind. After one month, that period extended itself to about one hour.

Now, I'm absolutely fine as long as I avoid all signs of her fairylike presence. I'm still waiting for the remnants of these crazy feelings for her to die, but I've existed the dark phase. *The worst is over*, and I couldn't be more relieved.

B). <u>RACHEL:</u> Red Flags Precede Revelations

I met a man on a dating app. Normally I struggle to connect with people, but after discovering a couple of big coincidences in our lives, I felt really aligned with him. We finally met after a month of constant texting and **I was hooked from then on**. I'd never felt anything like it before - he was just intoxicating. I wanted to define the relationship quite quickly, but he said he wanted to take things slowly, as he'd been hurt in the past. That filled me with anxiety. Things didn't add up from the start, but I needed him so I *ignored* **every single red flag** he was waving in my face.

The seven months we were together was the best and worst time of my life. When I knew I'd be seeing him soon or he was with me, I was euphoric, on cloud nine. When he was distant and ignoring my messages, however, I'd be so anxious that I couldn't function. He was on my mind 24/7, going over conversations, rehearsing future interactions, reading messages so often that I remembered them word for word. I was **living in a fantasy world** in my head – just *obsessed*. I used to spend hours staring at my phone, watching him go on and off WhatsApp without reading my messages. I spent a lot of my days crying, and using the private detective skills that I'd suddenly developed to see what he was up to online.

I started smoking weed every night soon after I met him, as it was the only way I could get myself to sleep. I became withdrawn from family and friends, and struggled to look after my young children. After too many things not adding up, I discovered that his 'ex', the mother of his child, who he saw and stayed with regularly, wasn't his ex. **I knew it was coming, but it still floored me.** He'd been lying and gaslighting me the whole time. She got rid of him and he blocked me. I spent a long time trying to get in touch. I sent emails he ignored, and even created fake Instagram accounts to message him from that he just constantly blocked. I left him voicemails until he changed his number. I feel so ashamed and embarrassed about my behaviour, but I was completely desperate. I don't like the person I've become. I used to feel relatively normal but now I feel crazy, and that's a really tough pill to swallow. I'm withdrawn, irritable, depressed, and find life overwhelming and pointless.

It's been a year since the split and I feel like I'm in hell. I cry and battle suicidal thoughts most days. Some days I have complete meltdowns. **Rationally, I can see he's not a good man, but I can't feel it.** It's as though it doesn't matter, because I need him. Everything reminds me of him, and I mean everything. My brain can create a connection anywhere, and there's no escape. I was fairly happy before I met him and now it feels like I'm trapped in a nightmare that I can't wake up from. I feel like I'm screaming all the time but no one can hear me, and it's the most terrifying thing when you can't see a way out. It's a lonely, isolating place to be, because it makes no sense, so who would understand unless you've experienced it? No one. So I keep it all inside, or just speak to others online who understand what I'm going through.

I'm literally trying everything I can think of to get over this. I've read everything I can find on limerence, I've started a psychology degree so I can one day study it for myself, I've had 3 different therapists, I'm on a million different supplements, I'm on antidepressants which I'm currently trying to come off, I've improved my diet as I read about the gut-brain connection, I've bought 27,000 self-help books, and I've looked into lucid dreaming to heal trauma. I've never felt such desperation to feel better.

I often find my brain scrambling for ways to hold on. Hoping that maybe, just maybe, we'll meet again one day and things will be different. It's hard to let go when I'm battling my own stubborn mind. I've been told that it's a choice; that I can choose to change my perspective; that I can choose to live in the moment and be happy, but the rumination can't just be switched off. Even when I'm focused on other things, he's there, waiting for a weak moment to take hold again. If I could choose happiness I would. This is not a choice, it's a curse.

I hate him and everything that he's done, but I need him. I'd go to the ends of the earth for him. I'm an addict and he is my drug.

NOTE FROM AUTHOR: This individual is clearly still limerent, and painfully so. Despite being highly astute, and proactive in her attitude towards recovery, she is struggling to 'free' herself from these emotions. She's well aware that her LO's personality is problematic in many ways, but still 'feels' that she needs him. Fortunately, however, having such **a decisive inner 'knowing'** that limerence is illusory and not 'real love' is a great position to be in. It's almost always what precedes true recovery (after which you no longer think about your LO, or *any* LOs).

This holds true even if you are *logically* aware of the damaging, superficial nature of a limerent bond, but still *viscerally* crave your LO. You see, this **inner, conscious <u>resolution</u>** to overcome limerence is exactly what will inspire you to do the proper psychological self-work that will enable you to truly <u>feel and act differently</u> (and permanently 'unstick' yourself from this pattern). The reprogramming described in this book (involving visualisation, affirmations and self-concept shifts) speaks to your subconscious mind *through emotion* and rewires it. I am confident that this individual will free herself in a matter of weeks once she starts to approach recovery in this way.

Ironically, recovering from limerence is so much more simple than we often make it out to be, yet at times, very unintuitive – above all, it requires faith that you can heal, and that your brain can (and inevitably will) change in response to the potent techniques that you now know how to employ.

C). <u>CHRIS</u>: Goal-Oriented Madness, Pain & Clarity

I'm Chris. I grew up in a loving but poor family – in a traditional Christian environment. My father was always away working. In his spare time, he mainly kept himself occupied behind his computer.

I always had to adhere to my parents' strict, religious rules, often feeling that what I wanted as an individual was of no real importance. None of them listened to me, let alone understood my feelings. To put it bluntly, other things were always more important: religion, money, and my siblings who spoke up more while I kept my struggles to myself. But, they did their best.

When I was 12, we moved house. I was forced to leave all of my friends behind, and became very lonely during puberty. With my family's oppressive attitude and my lack of companionship at school, I felt lost. The old family computer became my haven – I routinely escaped into it, eventually stumbling across some individuals with whom I felt I resonated by pure chance. They sent one another pirated games and music as expressions of friendship, and warmly accepted me into their motley crew. We generally bonded over our isolation and our shared love for technology and music, staying in touch for quite some time.

That little circle formed a big part of my social life during puberty, my 'escape'. I felt I could breathe amongst them – a creative, slightly rogue bunch of kids who lived to bend the rules and compete with one another. Besides them, I also found some more conventional friends with whom I started to routinely drop by a warm, all-inclusive rock/grunge club. It was there that I met the woman to whom I'm married today.

When my time at school came to a close, **I decided to study mathematics** at a nearby university, one renowned for its brutal difficulty. My final year was particularly tough, and my grades dipped unprecedentedly low despite me having given it my all. There was also a change in management that year, and I remember the new management just feeling 'wrong' to me – incongruent with the university's values. And I wasn't wrong; two years after I graduated, they shut the place down. It wasn't generating enough money, they claimed.

Since my parents were financially challenged, I felt as though I ought to have another crack at it. I needed to turn things around, that same year. The only shot I had at passing the year was by acing the oral re-sit exams. I studied for all I was worth, finally answering all of the questions flawlessly and finishing with a full board of Firsts.

At that time, I felt very insecure about myself. Having received very poor marks for the best part of the year had really chipped away at my self-esteem. I also disliked how much university life distanced me from the impartial, judgment-free **realm of computers**, which had very much come to represent a safe haven for me.

But, **I dived right into a PhD**, also in mathematics; I couldn't not, as my mind was begging me to keep going… imploring me to delve deeper and deeper into the abstract, logical world of numbers. I felt liberated from human constraints and capricious emotions when I was allowed to bask in the mathematical headspace, undisturbed. To cut a long story short, I ended up having a revelation in my second year – despite having always imagined myself working in industry, I felt an inexorable urge propelling me towards the world of academia. The idea of being valued for the contents of my mind, and my ability to impart them to others, was highly appealing to me. I allowed myself to continue down the trajectory I was on and became an Assistant Professor in the year 2000.

This required that I move across the country. While I had just started seriously dating my current significant other (SO), the job offer was a golden ticket – one that I couldn't refuse.

And so I went for it, and we left. I felt liberated from my family, and their religious ways. Couldn't wait to launch myself towards work that brought me closer to my natural state.

My SO, on the other hand, does not share my affinity for daring action or self-development. Moving was a huge issue for her, but she did it in the end. She was afraid of losing me, and her fears just about outweighed the downsides in her head. It did prove a tricky transition for her - she has since struggled to blend in, make new friends, grow new roots. This has caused her a lot of pain and frustration, and lead to her battling what has morphed into chronic depression.

I adore academia. The way I see it, it's really about people interacting, sharing ideas, and eventually *synchronising and aligning*.

One day, we were visited by another university – fresh faces to connect with and bounce ideas off. **That was when I first saw her, my redhead**. She was engrossed in her work, and I wasn't plucky enough to introduce myself. I just grabbed a coffee and went back to my desk. But even now, nine years later, I remember how potently her presence affected me that day. Something primitive and deeply rooted inside me just *drew a big arrow towards her*. Now, I know to refer to that as the infamous limerent 'glimmer' – illusory, delusional, but oh so hard to avoid falling for when you aren't aware that doing so will drag you to hell and back.

"That one redhead chick was hot", I commented to my friend, but he didn't understand – apparently, her blonde friend was far more attractive. But, I knew better.

The visitors left and were forgotten, and life went on. My SO went to the psychologist and was diagnosed with chronic depression. Her gloomy moods had always affected and worried me ... but suddenly, it felt like they were Here To Stay. That her depression was going to define my life. I felt betrayed by it, and by her. But I tried to be loyal. Tried to help her. Tried to stay by her side.

A few years later, the visitors returned as randomly as they had appeared the first time. I was sitting at my desk when the redhead introduced herself to me. She came up to me, and complimented my hair. We instantly connected - every word she spoke fitted perfectly with mine. Flawless synchronisation. **To say we hit it off does it injustice**.

It was summer, so we agreed to go for lunchtime walks during her stay. We'd shoot each other a message and meet at the building's entrance. Seeing her smile upon seeing me was magical. Oh, we'd talk for hours and tease each other... throwing witty remarks back and forth. I remember feeling 'drugged', and far from my normal, guarded self, even throwing in sexual innuendo (albeit covertly enough to be subtle). She loved it.

She smoked and didn't take care of herself. Bizarrely, I felt inspired to take care of her... in an almost fatherly fashion. Which is, well, not the standard type of thing I do for colleagues. We just really hit it off. This transitioned into us chatting outside of work, over WhatsApp. Just funny little jokes, little more. Felt really wonderful though.

On her last day, I remember feeling undeniably gloomy; what had been so fun was about to end. I remember booking an extra hour off work, just to be with her until her ride arrived to bring her back to the airport.

When we were waiting for the taxi there, in the sun, she started to ramble on about her problems with her love life and past lovers. That must've been a hint, right? I mean, why else would you tell someone you really hit it off with about these sorts of things?

I felt butterflies in my stomach, but believed that it was just a one-off – just some fun, and some mental stimulation. I shrugged it off; life goes on, right? I had no clue what was in store for me... that those feelings would morph into something much worse, and of grotesque, colossal dimensions.

After she left, we kept in touch via WhatsApp. I stressed that she really ought to kick her smoking habit – that it was bad for her. Of course, we flirted too. Just witty remarks and a few puns – I like to mess around with people's train of thought, that's just me. Made sure my SO never saw the messages, of course...

This woman, who we can now call my **former limerent object** (FLO), is a very caring person – probably the most empathetic, emotionally perceptive person I know. And I think those are wonderful virtues. One day, she received some tragic news about a close university friend of hers. I wanted to cheer her up – to send her an emergency package with all kinds of things to be opened only in case of emergency, e.g. if she needed to be cheered up. I made that box and ordered the gifts, while my SO remained oblivious. She had no clue about the existence of my FLO, nor about what was going on in my head. Of course, I felt guilty for the secrecy.

We kept in touch, she and I. It was a warm, mostly 'platonic' connection at the time. When she returned to my home country to conduct some research, I shuffled my schedule to be able to be with her during her lunch break. I remember the two of us sitting together alone, while the rest of her team sat at another table.

After this second little stint together, we once again returned to our normal work, and normal lives. Lost contact.

Around this time, my SO and I were struggling, badly. I was stressed with work, and naturally, her mental health left a lot to be desired. She was in a dark place and couldn't cope. But, I was starting to see that I could **no longer be her sole source of happiness** – that she needed to learn how to get *herself* out of slumps. Screaming fights ensued, involving her shouting in front of the kids that we 'needed a divorce'. I felt us being closed in by an abyss… a dark pit.

But, I crawled out of it, slowly. Every day, I ensured to do things that gave me energy. I went to the gym, lifted weights and rowed. Of course, I found myself **thinking about my redhead**. Wondering how she was, fantasising about seeing her again. Goodness, I could no longer lie to myself - she had made such an impression on me.

Months passed, and slowly but surely, I crawled out of that dismally dark place. My relationship with my SO was abysmal and I was strongly considering divorce. But, I knew that I needed to give my children a better youth than the one I'd had. They're so important to me, and my connection with them is beautiful. I found myself horribly conflicted. I sought the advice of a psychologist, as well as a confidential counsellor from work. They both suggested that I divorce my SO as soon as possible. But I didn't – couldn't do it to the kids.

So, my SO and I then entered an equilibrium of sorts. We weren't warm or jovial with each other, but we got by and worked as a team.

Soon, we learnt that she suffered from other disorders as well as depression. Frankly, it all felt like a death sentence and changed how I perceived her. She felt worthless too, even going as far as to tell me that she'd understand if I had a mistress. Said that love, in itself, was not enough in a relationship. I only perceived her to be devaluing herself by speaking like this, and *her passivity irritated me*. She was practically giving me a free pass to explore things outside our relationship.

It was months later that I once again saw my FLO in person. I was desperate to know where I stood with her. Was it all in my head? But, I made sure not to pack any condoms when I prepared my suitcase for the trip. **I wanted to be as objective as possible**, and any stupid ideas in my head would have been sure to mess up my objectivity. Plus, *nothing was going to happen*. As soon as I had arrived at my hotel, I let her know I was there. We teased each other a bit over WhatsApp, and a few minutes later, she met me outside the building.

To see her again, to hug her and breathe in her scent... Wow.

The days we spent together, I worked very productively – I had prepared well. And during my lunch breaks and in the evenings, I had time with my redhead. One evening, she asked me something that didn't make any sense to me at the time. *Had I fallen in love recently*?

I mean, she knew I was married, didn't she? That's an impertinent question to ask under those circumstances, right? But, maybe she felt the tension too, and wanted clarity? I told her that there was *that one redhead* who had never really exited my head. It was as if she'd waited for that cue – she grabbed my hand, folded it into mine, and smiled knowingly. Holding hands like that implied that she understood the feelings that she had unleashed in me. I was jittery, **teeth clattering uncontrollably, arms and legs shaking**, while we walked back to my hotel room.

I told her I had some treats for her, stashed away in my luggage. Asked her to wait outside my hotel room, while I dug around and fetched them. Thank goodness I hadn't packed the condoms – things could have got messy. I brought her the sweets and held her in my arms, breathing in her scent. I gave her a kiss on her forehead, wishing her a good night. **It was tough to leave her.** But I returned to my room feeling validated.

We went out for lunch again the next day, and she brought me to a delicious pasta place. At the restaurant's entrance, she whispered in my ear that **she knew what she'd do to me,** if only there were no people around. My eyes opened wide when I assimilated what she'd said, but we were already being guided to our table by the waitress. Plus, I still had no condoms on me.

...

She didn't order *anything*. Claimed she wasn't hungry – I knew she had a problematic relationship with food. I ordered a steak sandwich, which was probably the best one I had ever eaten. Shared my fries with her, insisting she ate a few. She started caressing my wedding ring, flashing me the odd intense, piercing look paired with a smile. It was the most sexual thing I had ever experienced.

We had fun, joked around, shared anecdotes – at last, some real, quality time together. She told me **she had always wanted to be a writer**, but had picked another career path for economic reasons. That it was still her dream to one day pursue that. She also told me how she experimented with hallucinogens while young, describing how the world had distorted around her and how amusing it had been. That I found really jarring, as I'm pretty much completely against drugs.

We said our goodbyes and I went home. The first thing I did at the airport was write to her to tell her that I already missed her. She told me not to 'be so simple about it'. I didn't fully comprehend her at the time. Did she mean I should've worded it more elegantly? That the crass directness of those commonly overused words clashed with my otherwise complex personality... with our complex connection?

Well, that was it – I was, once again, home with my SO. My chronically depressed, co-dependent, OCD-leaning SO, who was demonstrating herself to be incapable of making new friends and growing new roots. Who wasn't playful and teasing... who didn't radiate sexuality and desire. Who was familiar, colourless, bland.

I sent message after message to my LO. I touched on that evening at the hotel – about the things I'd felt, and about my shitty marriage. Told her I needed time to work on things, that I needed to go NC to figure out my life.

It was then that I reached a shaky conclusion – I had to divorce my SO. It just made sense. So I told her I wanted out. When she asked me if it was about my trip abroad, **about that redhead** (who I had, by this point, mentioned to her in passing), I replied with a firm 'no'. I mean, nothing had actually happened between my FLO and I, right? This was just me realising that, after our fights and evident dissipating interest in each other, enough was enough, right? But, I nonetheless decided to tell her what had happened in front of the hotel. That I had had the chance to do things that weren't okay, but hadn't.

Surprisingly, my SO was understanding – the past years had been undeniably rough for us both. Instead of fuming at me, she looked me in the eyes and asked for a second chance. Asked for us to try partner therapy, before we decided that the situation was *beyond remedy.*

I agreed, and we went to an EFT couples' therapist.

In a haze, I unleashed my innermost feelings, blurting out that all I wanted was for my SO to support my dreams. Explained how driven and passionate I am, and how important challenging myself and growing in my field is to me. How I was eager to practice coding on the side. How I wanted my SO to be able to stand up to me, to debate with me... and, how I also missed intimacy in our relationship.

My SO remained half-frozen, but our therapist understood me. It was crystal clear to her that my SO was the intransigent one who needed to change. I told her that I was infuriated and upset – **I had desperately wanted a soulmate**, to be understood in life, and to have a deep connection to someone who was on the same wavelength as me. Instead, I had ended up with someone who froze up and wasn't strong. But, we slowly seemed to come to an understanding, ending on a good note.

Then COVID hit the world. My SO and I very much fell into our own routines. I worked remotely from the kitchen, while she looked after the kids during that time (her work closed). But with the kids at home, on top of memories of me saying that I 'needed things' in the relationship (to which my SO mentally added 'or else it is divorce'), she once again started to despair. The things she had wanted to do as part of our therapy talks couldn't be done due to COVID, and she felt insufficient and uneasy.

To add insult to injury, she began developing unrealistic fears - every day, something else popped up and petrified her. This irrationality seemed extremely weak to me, adding to the **enormous heap of shortcomings** I already saw in her.

During this surreal quarantine period, I reached out to my FLO. We chatted more about my dreams; I told her that I wanted to study more, also encouraging her to follow her own passions. If the elephant's too big, cut it into pieces. Just write a few hundred words every day, I told her. Keep it achievable – I broke my work down into chunks too, after all. I truly wanted to inspire her, to be a positive influence to my redhead.

Our conversations became a routine, and one I loved. My studies progressed well. She later confessed that I had roused her motivation, too – it **felt like we were reconnecting**. Until she mentioned how overwhelmed she'd been feeling recently, and how she'd done 'some stupid things to feel alive.' Unsure *where exactly* she was going, I cautiously confessed that I understood why people do such things. You can only be locked up for so long, right? Totally get it.

I prompted her further the next day, until she told me that she had been sleeping with a random guy who she felt 'understood the depths of her pain.'

Cheating on her SO. *Okay.* I told her that she was, indeed, being self-destructive. That it wouldn't help her in the long run, and to please be careful. Some doors you don't want to open, some roads you don't want to wander down. *The brain remembers, and paths trodden will be used more often.* I forced myself to go NC again, and deleted all of our chat history. Saddened but determined, I continued on with my studies, very much alone in life.

Months later, it dawned on me that I liked being in contact with my FLO more than I resented her indiscretion and impulsivity. After all, I wasn't her SO, was I? So, I had no right to judge her.

I reinstalled WhatsApp.

She told me that her **mother had been diagnosed with pancreatic cancer** - that things were looking grim. And me, trying to be a good friend, shakingly typed simple, positive things to cheer her up. She forwarded me some of her poetry, and I had actually written some too (which turned out much, much better than I had expected). Staying true to our brand, we jokingly teased each other again. I encouraged her to look after herself and sent her a stream of idiotic memes. I soon put the brakes on my messaging, because I wasn't getting much back from her – plus, there's a certain delicacy required when you're supporting someone going through hell. You need to be tactful – the idea is to help after all, right?

After a few weeks of silence, I got another message from her. She wasn't in a good place. I tried to tell her to take better care of her own needs, too. Tried to tell her that 'this too shall pass'. I, of all people, *knew* what she was going through, able to clearly envision her in **a personal abyss**. I knew what it was like to hit the floor and dwell there. But I wanted her to be able to brave it with a friend, instead of suffering in solitude as I had. After all, I only wanted to be a good friend to her, right? (Right?)

She started to tell me that she missed the walks with me, and missed me in general. I replied that *I missed her so much* that it had physically hurt me over the past year. And that I felt like the world made sense again... that I was warm inside. Our conversation underwent a brusque change of course that evening. She told me how she was proud of me, and of how passionate I was. Proud of how I always supported her in pursuing her dreams.

We also spoke about that evening in the hotel – about how hard it had been to be good. She took it a step further, typing **how wonderful it would be to have sex**. I replied that, in retrospect, we should've just gone for it back then. I mean, it wasn't like it had been a great year, you know.

I told her that I had previously cut contact because *she got too deep under my skin*, yet how I once again felt more aligned with her than ever. How not a week went by when she wasn't in my mind. She said that she didn't want to break apart my 'cute family', and that maybe it was best that we don't spend too much time together, because *we always ended up 'here'*. I told her that I had <u>seriously wanted a divorce</u> earlier on, and that after this year, I'd pull through with it. And how my SO was okay with me having a mistress. After a whole lot more sexual innuendo, we agreed to go to bed and, erhm, sleep.

We tried to spend as much time online as we could. We'd share stupid jokes, and little snippets of things we came across. It felt as though we'd confessed mutual feelings, even though we hadn't explicitly done so.

And at that time, that was fine by me. I mean, she had other things to worry about, with her mom and COVID. She was the one in *the abyss*. I, on the other hand, was just there to cheer her up. I could figure out what it all meant afterwards. Naturally, she was gloomy throughout our talks, but I knew her situation must be putting a dark filter on things, right? I mean, her mom's state was only deteriorating. She talked about her problems from the past, and I shared my stories as well. I tried to bond with her... Tried to nudge her into a slightly more positive frame of mind. Tried to provide her with the mental stimulation that *I had always wanted* while stuck in *my own* abyss.

And whenever she was overly cynical, I parried her, gently but assuredly pointing at the flaws of her reasoning. *Teasingly*. We had **deep philosophical discussions** - the ones I just craved. I enjoyed it so, so much. Even though she came across as really dark and grim at times – and why wouldn't she be considering her situation – she just understood me perfectly. She told me that she had wanted to die earlier on, and I confessed that I had sensed that. I told her that was why I was bugging her all the time. Told her that **we obviously needed each other to *thrive* in life**. That I wanted to be there for her.

Her spirits lifted a little at one point, and she felt like celebrating with me. Told me she had a really great unopened whiskey and wanted to toast to the end of the abyss. It started off safe enough (I toasted to her health, and to crawling out of the pit she had fallen into while trying to alleviate her mother's pain), but *boy, did it derail*.

I ended up confessing that I truly did want to be there for her, as much as I realistically could be. She told me that she loved talking to me, but that she also **wondered if it did me harm**. She said she apologised if it did, because she greatly admired me for being the dad I am. Insinuated that my SO must be wonderful, too.

At that point, I felt a lump in my throat – she was referring to the life I had and didn't want, and in doing so, she was making it feel all the more real. When what I *actually* wanted was *a life with her,* however absurd and inappropriate that desire was. I almost told her that I was keen to burn all bridges with my SO, because **I felt connected to her, *my redhead*, instead**. In turn, she told me about her past relationship troubles, and about some questionable, intimate things that I promised I'd keep to myself.

When I was properly intoxicated, I risked telling her that I *figured we were compatible*. She teased back that it may have also crossed her mind, adding that she'd never admit it. I replied that the best I could do was to make sure that she, my redhead, thrived in life. **I told her I loved her**. She replied that it was probably only because I was emotionally 'available'. No, I told her, one of the few things I was sure of was that I wanted her in my life. That I had been trying for the last seven years to have her in it. She replied that she felt that **we'd have an overly incendiary effect** on each other's life. That she really didn't want anything, because she had given up on romance.

I told her that I didn't want to force anything, but that my feelings were genuine. She confirmed that they must be, because of the effect I had on her. It was obvious when we spoke, and even more so when we saw each other in person. That comment seemed to clash wholeheartedly with her **previous renouncement of love** – trying to decipher her intentions was infuriating.

Bringing me back to reality, she went on to mention that 'some things change when you actually live them'. That the sacrifices that you need to make to live them out can make you resent the other person… that it's often best to **leave some adventures in Dreamland,** where everything's perfect. I disagreed with her resoundingly. She told me that she wanted to be there for me too, but did not want to cause me any pain. I told her not to worry, admitting to her that my life was entirely empty without her.

She told me she wanted to go back to her SO again, to which I replied that – no matter what – she could return to me. That I'd wait for her. (In retrospect, I can't believe how 'drugged' on limerent emotions I was – how unaware I was that my boundaries had fallen flat, and that my dignity had dissolved)…

I finally drunkenly confessed it: that **I would throw it all away for her**. She told me she didn't want to know, and had always sensed that we were trouble together. And I asked her… *Trouble, or just a genuine match?* She couldn't respond.

But, she did know that she wanted to visit my region when the COVID restrictions relaxed a bit. And spend time with me. She told me that she found the way I challenged her irresistible. I told her she was worth challenging. **She had always known how I felt**, she admitted, since we'd met. *How nice it'd be if things were simple.* We ended our messaging on an undeniably romantic note that evening. She admitted that she missed it so much – **that me-specific feeling** – before apologising for being tired and incoherent.

The next morning, I told her I was glad to have it in the open. Tired of hiding and running. But that I knew that she needed to first focus on herself – the rest could truly wait.

Well, our back-and-forth communication continued. We shared our ideas and feelings with zero inhibitions, unmistakeably bonding. I told her about all of my problems with my SO, and she opened up more about her past relationship issues. About that one guy who still seemed to have an emotional hold on her, and who she'd always go on about. About how she'd never managed to find a 'good relationship'. I asked her, **what about trying again, with someone who *gets you*?**

She conceded that she probably did need to see a therapist. Before then, she'd always flat-out rejected the suggestion. It felt like we were finally progressing – an enormous victory. In my head, it felt like the first step of that master plan of mine to get her over here. Not as a mistress, but as a new SO.

But, she told me that she couldn't leave her SO. Because they functioned. It wasn't her dream, but it was what she needed, she claimed. To have more than that, a partner in crime, someone who understands and challenges you, she said, was '**a dream that she could no longer believe in**'.

I didn't know what to say to that, but dared to reply that spending time with her *felt like breathing*. She said it did for her as well. I said I'd be fighting tooth and nail to keep doing it. That I couldn't fathom stopping. She replied that 'it sounded like a drug, put like that'... that she might, after all, be bad for me. And if I felt that she was, she'd respect that. But that it's rare to find someone so mentally and spiritually aligned with you.

I told her I didn't want her to cheat on her SO for me. Because, despite, you know, us having an obvious emotional affair, intercourse is one of those boundaries. It just **wouldn't fit my**

moral framework. According to an earlier remark from my FLO, I 'still' harboured 'some pretty rigid ideas of right and wrong' which, at times, 'constituted my own prison.'

But, she ironically ended up telling me to focus on healing my relationship with my SO. Indignant, I explained back that I didn't want to do that – that my marriage was beyond repair. There was an insistent voice in my head telling me that it really wasn't that bad, wondering why I was even being so emphatic. But, I mainly felt devastated because the bubble around me was bursting; I was being reminded of what my FLO and I really were (nothing).

The next morning, she apologised. Confessed that the effect I had on her was wild, but that she was aware no one could fix her. That *that* was why she was so cold and cerebral at times. But, that she nonetheless *still* found herself thinking of all the fun things we could do together... of how it would be to make love. That she wanted to be a part of my life *in a way that wouldn't hurt me*. And that if I thought that talking to her was detrimental to my mental health, we could take steps back. Ended up saying that I really helped her through her lowest days.

We hopped back and forth in this weird, intricate dance of ours for days. One moment, we'd be bonding and telling each other how wonderful we were, and **how committed we were to solving this damn puzzle** of ours with regards to our personal lives/SOs. The next, however, she'd abruptly switch state, presenting as eerily sensible and trying to put a brake on things for 'fear of hurting me' – talk about subjecting me to *intermittent reward cycles*. I'd tell her not to do that. Then, she'd admit that she did really like me, and that our connection 'was like a strong stimulant drug', or, more accurately, how she'd imagine one to feel.

It was maddening. To be encapsulated in such an all-consuming, tangible, as-real-as-can-be connection, yet feel it slipping out of your hands the *whole* time. The uncertainty, and unclarity of it all – just maddening.

At one point, she raised a topic that we had previously skimmed over. I had told her that before my SO, I had fallen in love with someone else, someone who impacted me intensely back then. I'd told her that I have this type: 'foreign', and 'hot'. My FLO playfully added 'with issues', to which I wrote 'who's gifted at helping others'. That woman was also someone with whom I felt the same kind of overpowering attraction. She had suffered sexual abuse as a child, and had ended up working as a psychologist helping rape victims. She and I ended up as friends, although I had initially wanted more.

Before educating myself on limerence, I had learnt to **appreciate that glimmer**. It was a Good Thing, right? I guess it is, but in moderation and under certain circumstances. You see, I also experienced a type of glimmer sensation when I met the best platonic friend I made in my youth – he was a great guy, but thoroughly broken inside as well. But, someone who really helped me battle against my loneliness when I was in real need of a friend. Eventually, we went our separate ways, but I'll always remember him and our special bond fondly.

But looking back, I realise that I always considered the glimmer Profoundly Good and, importantly, Real… and incapable of inducing harm. No one told me otherwise, and all the movies were based on it, right? So I assumed it was just one of those things that everyone experienced – that, and the **neurochemical madness** that follows it (when it is a **Romantic Glimmer**, of course) – but I was wrong.

I realised I was still, at points, evading the truth and ignoring the obvious with regards to my problematic feelings. I wanted to change things this time, and vowed to not delete my chat history anymore. It was better that I processed it all rather than running away. What's more, deleting it felt like erasing a part of me that I didn't *want* to erase. I now understood how she felt about me, and was committed to doing things differently. To processing my feelings, rather than burying them.

My FLO explained that she's prone to opening up to guys and expecting them to be her therapists, when she should really seek professional help herself. How that **makes them fall in love with her**, complicating things even more… how that was a real pattern with her. And that it wasn't fair, because I wasn't a therapist and she shouldn't be burdening me with all of her trauma.

Of course, I responded by assuring her it *didn't* feel like therapy or burden me, because it was really about us both – two people mutually opening up. That she was an equal, not a psychological case to assess and resolve. That there's this human thing called 'emotional vulnerability', and that it's needed for connectedness and fulfilment in life.

"Yeah, but a part of me expects you to stay objective. Which I know isn't realistic or possible"... (Looking back, I remember this moment. My brain ironically interpreted this line as a cue to become even more obsessive, despite the severity of the situation starting to dawn on me. Sigh...)

My FLO was, at that point in time, upset with me for having confessed my feelings to my SO. She didn't want to hear that I had... didn't want to negatively impact the lives of others. Wanted to call me in person to talk about it after five minutes.

But, those five minutes lapsed into an hour. And since she had stood me up in the past, I... didn't know what to expect. So, I sent her my earlier-prepared goodbye note. In it, I mostly told her about how I enjoyed connecting with her, but understood we'd no **longer be available to each other** in the future – told her that she needed to focus more on herself and go into proper therapy. That I'd kick her SO's a** if he didn't support her in the future.

I also added that she'd need to pick a role to assign to me. I was *either* her therapist, her friend, or... well... you know. But I don't switch back and forth between roles.

She eventually did phone me back, and we spoke some more. And as soon as she started to intentionally meander, I attempted to steer her back towards what she had previously intended to ask me. I told her about the ramifications of that earlier visit, involving us standing by the hotel room. That my SO had asked me a direct question, and that I'm not a lying type – **I give direct answers**. That she'd discovered something was going on, even though nothing physical had actually happened.

During the phone call, I asked her directly if she HAD feelings for me. If something WAS going on. After asking her twice, she broke, and hoarsely told me that she had, indeed, **fallen in love with me**. To me, this felt like the moment I had been waiting for all these years. I reassured her that my relationship with my SO was nothing to do with her, and that it was breaking down, anyway. Told her that what I really wanted to do was sit down with her and figure out what *we could do* in the future, together.

When our conversation came to an end, my FLO burst into tears, saying that she didn't want to go home to her SO. Got me crying, too.

To me, this was a **really pivotal moment**. She would be stuck in her family's apartment for one more day before she returned home, but right there and then, it felt like *promises had really been made*. The next day, I told my FLO that I was in low power mode but with the added bonus of fluttering sensations, wanting to hear her voice, and feeling like a bit of an idiot.

I, at that time, was writing a tonne – predominantly about how my marriage was doomed and I needed to bail from it. However, later that same day, my redhead FLO seemed to be all of a sudden intent on trying to **coax me to work on it**. She started to speak similarly reasonably about her own relationship. Said she wanted to reinvent the relationship *on her terms,* so that it made sense to her.

With regards to how she envisioned the future, she almost seemed to have <u>forgotten the conversation </u>we had had earlier that day... and the promises that had been made. She eventually just point-blank told me that being with her **was out of the question**, because of the way relationships had made her feel in the past. She told me that she'd either mould her current relationship into what she wanted it to be, or decide to stay alone. That she wouldn't be able to 'respect herself' otherwise...

I remember how something **just *snapped* inside of me** back then. Something inside of me started *screaming*, slowly and softly at first, but increasing in volume. I noticed I wasn't as sharp and witty as I had been in the previous weeks, when I had been floating on a cloud of dopamine and possibilities. I also wasn't being as nice to my FLO. In fact, *I told her she had a pretty skewed idea of love* – in light of her earlier remarks, our phone call, and her stolen confession. In light of how I felt that she played with me, toyed with me, pulled the rug from under me. I really felt hurt.

At this point, she returned to where her SO and friends live – told me to expect some radio silence. I felt utterly alone.

Now that I knew she'd be 'getting space', and that she was outside of the pressure cooker she had previously been locked inside (giving me guaranteed access to her time and attention), I *just* felt … lost.

The next morning, however, she contacted me again. After a while, she decided to talk to me about my earlier remarks on love. She told me I had no idea about her idea of love. That my 'vast experience of one relationship' wasn't enough to make a comment, and that I sometimes needed to be put in my place... I even ended up apologising to her, although I still knew I had a point. I failed to provide her with any of my regular responses. Felt downbeat, and unnaturally sluggish. I was crashing, badly.

I was making a conscious effort to ease my vigour a little – to be less open, to stop leaving **all of my cards scattered** on the table. I just needed to make sense of my emotions, because by that point, they were bouncing off the ceiling. Tried to be more objective, and distanced myself emotionally. We still chatted, but not so intimately. But, the **screaming in my head** became less and less tolerable.

Soon, she asked me how I was doing. I told her that I had become introspective, wanting to process the weird things I had been feeling (and typing) in hazy, drunken states. That I wanted to learn from my mistakes, rather than continually repeating them. And that I been speaking with my SO about what I need in a relationship (in truth, I was actually trying to torpedo   my   marriage   at   that   point   in   time).

The screaming was fast becoming unbearable.

But, my FLO was her usual cheerful, quirky self, chattering away about everything she was up to. Telling me that I needed to be careful about **labelling what I learnt about myself** in my introspections. That I should be kind to myself while I reflected, because I'm very intense when it comes to feelings, to which she added a destabilising, '*as am I*.' She wrote that we sometimes need to 'recharge our batteries', because long-term relationships come with a lot of frustrations. That it's normal and healthy to have needs, and these needs can take on different forms. That we sometimes need to fall in love in order to feel hope again.

I told her that something at the back of my head was going off... telling me that all the pieces of the puzzle were somehow laid out on the table. That it was just a feeling, but one that I had learnt to listen to. **That tingling that precedes clarity**... that tranquil void where things eventually start to make sense.

I told her that **I don't generally fall in love,** *so when I do, I need to 'get it'*. Poetically stated that I was going through a stimulant-like withdrawal, trying to desperately piece the puzzle together.

It was then that I first truly started to piece together what was hurting my LO. I'm everything but a psychologist, but this is what I made of it:

*Narcissistic mother, absent father. Was a scapegoat for her mother, while her brother was the golden child. Lonely youth. Textbook case of **instrumental parentification**, involving her being responsible for all household duties at a very young age. Father became ill – during his illness, mother had affair. **Emotional parentification**: mother irresponsibly shared intimate details and lacked empathy.*

*Co-dependent relationship with that one ex-boyfriend, who still represents a **gold standard** to her. Relationship ended because he felt obliged to return back to former girlfriend to repay a debt. There were also prior cases where he abandoned her – promised to be there forever, but wasn't able to be. He later developed damaging habits to numb his pain, which troubled her immensely. Shortly afterwards, her father died. She dealt with additional stress at school, and she wasn't able to pursue her dreams because of her family's financial situation. Picked up smoking as a coping mechanism.*

*Extremely caring and empathetic nature. Does not **adhere to traditional boundaries** for platonic relationships, enmeshing with all the individuals closest to her. Current relationship with her SO does not come close to fulfilling her emotional needs – leaves her starving. She considers it a dull, safe haven. But, still needs to 'do crazy things' in order to breathe. Has developed a pattern where she falls into intense emotional affairs, which are rapidly curtailed by her in a sudden attempt to 'normalise things'. Cycles featuring clear **extinction, resurgence behaviour**: no stable end situation.*

I pointed her towards 'parentification' as a first step. Didn't want to feed her too much, but hey, I wanted to help her. She thought it was really interesting that there was a term 'parentification', but failed to see *how it applied to her*. Claimed that labels, while useful in therapy, did not help her understand herself or others. I replied that I also wasn't one to put nice little tags on messy human things in order to stop thinking about them, if that's what she was hinting at. Labels don't define us, I continued, but they can point to **the existence of mental frameworks** that are constricting and limiting us.

That was when we started to mentally drift apart – to become *desynchronised*. I was frustrated that the constructive effort I was pouring into solving her problems wasn't being appreciated how it should've been – but then again, my strategy is to tear into things relentlessly until I get to the core of the issue. Not everyone can be expected to be on board with that.

She also objected to something I'd said about relationships: that it's your responsibility to take care of your SO, and make sure *their* emotional batteries are kept 'charged'. She thought it was a **very naïve outlook on love**, telling me that there's only time for that level of doting selflessness in high school.

I endured sleepless nights for days and days on end, and I was crashing. She noticed. Told me that she wanted me to find my happiness and relax. I told her not to worry about me… that she didn't need to help *me*. FLO: "Oh, that's what you think I'm doing? That's… I hope that's true."

We drifted further. I disagreed with her depiction of what a relationship was. I think two people in a relationship *have* to look out for each other. If you claim there's no time to maintain your relationship, you'll inevitably see it crumble. To that, I can attest.

Now feeling entirely out of sync with her, I told her I'd probably be offline for a while, or unresponsive. That I wanted to wrap up my fruitless overthinking and throw myself back into the land of living.

A day later, I tried to whip up and send her a few small sentences. Spent hours on them.

*I guess I have, in a way, wrapped up my excessive thinking. I need to end this weird Ouroboros cycle I've fallen into with you. I guess I understand it better now, why I acted the way I did, and why I felt the things I felt. But the 'understanding' itself won't prevent it from happening again, that I know. When we interact a lot, **something inside of me is stirred** that I can't really put into words.*

*The real problem is that, **subconsciously, I've never been able** to put you in the 'friend' category. And that probably will never change. I just can't be your friend. I'm sorry. I did try to be just-a-friend, but there's too much chemistry. And it gets me every time. I say stupid, heart-felt things. You then end up being the responsible one, which makes me feel bad. Slowing down the pace doesn't help either. **It just limits the playing time**, making it more fun the next time around.*

There are a lot of other angles and nuances here too, of course, but I've covered the core of the puzzle.

And she got angry with me. Apparently sensed it was coming – knew this was how I'd do it. Said she 'never expected anything from me anyway', if it was any consolation. Even though I insisted on telling her repeatedly that I wanted her in my life (and that I wanted to be there for her no matter what happens), she told me I was lucky she didn't believe it. That the only way to really end the cycle is to stop altogether, that she needed to keep her end of the bargain too. That she supported my decision and would ensure it didn't happen again. Screaming in my head was maximal. **Coherent thought was impossible**.

Over the course of the following night, I wrote:

Look, I'll be there for you ... If a crisis breaks out tomorrow or if you truly need me, I'll quit my whining and try to help you however I can, like I tried last time.

You know I want you in my life. Desperately. That's the whole problem.

I need to stop running in circles, though. Some things never were on the table and I need to accept that. I guess I misinterpret your cues and ignore what you literally say, sometimes reading things that aren't said... also maybe putting too much weight on the 'crazier' of our interactions. But those moments – they're stuck in my head. If you would, please answer one question for me. What is this thing that went on between us these last few years? Pretty sure we never intended a therapeutic relationship. :)

But, if this is a friendship, I don't get it either. Guess if it is, I really need to carefully rethink my boundaries, particularly about what I should be comfortable with sharing, and the attachment and connectedness I should allow myself to feel.

*What I tried to express earlier is that, to me, this has **never been a friendship**. I guess I'm mentally grieving. Because it feels like a crucial part of me has slipped away over these past few weeks. **I can't work, can't sleep. Can't eat.** I feel lost and miserable. And to top it all off, I'm really struggling to get my thoughts down on paper. These paragraphs have taken me hours. In reply to you 'knowing this would unfold in advance': Well, I guess I also knew full well that I'd end up feeling like this, when I was trying to support you... (No longer being able to eat was unexpected, though. Goodbye COVID kilos, I guess).*

*Tell you what, I want you to tell me one final time that you **honestly really think we've been nothing more than 'good friends'** all along... To explain to me, one more time, that I'm a fool. I need to hear it. I'll toughen this one out, and I will never talk about my feelings in this way ever again. I'll just be there when you need me. But, our interactions will need to transform, and quickly. I'll need you to play your part and help me in staying within these new boundaries.*

She was cold in response – said some hurtful, jarring things. "We're obviously not good friends, you're right. Good friends don't treat each other like poison." When I asked her what she wanted from me, or with me – **chemistry, deep interactions, light-heartedness** – she said "that's it… you just overreact to everything."

I thanked her, telling her that was precisely what I needed to hear. FLO: "Look, **I've always just enjoyed talking to you**. What you need to do is to learn to chill, to not get so caught up in your own head. You ruin nice things that come by, by submitting them to your mind grinder. So yeah, you're right, I can't be in your life. I'm too nice, too open, too permissive. I get people to open up and they think we have a special connection, but it's really about them. The depth, all of it. They're seeing a reflection of themselves – it's always the same."

Me: "No, it's not – you truly connect with them and it hits them hard." FLO: "Oh really? Do you really think *you're* sharp enough to see what's going on here, that you're different from the rest? I've been in thousands of situations like this."

Me: "It's not ALL about the people you connect with and *their* issues… their tendency to fall into strange dynamics with you. What's really going on here is about you. You're sending signs their way, of wanting a deep connection. There are signals that they're misreading – they get confused. And even if it *were* purely about them, at some point they'd want something back… **they'd want to be validated in their role**."

FLO: "Only the ones with the biggest ego would want to be validated." Me: "Only the ones that dare to open up and have hope, who dare to take a plunge." FLO: "There's no plunge to be taken – this is obsession and insecurity you're describing." Me: "Look, every human wants to be validated. But the real question here is, why didn't we adhere to **the friendship ruleset**, if what we have is truly so platonic?".

FLO: 'I'm not like you, okay. I don't need to constrain myself, or label and 'understand' everything… that's something about yourself that you need to fix, in my opinion. When you fixate on things too much, you're guaranteed to lose them. Plus, you're irritating me right now. I think its best if we just stop. I'm tired of feeling guilty and like I'm hurting you."

The next day, I wrote her a goodbye note.

I don't believe in forever, but I'll drop contact on my end. This'll be my last message.

I don't believe this can evolve into a healthy friendship. Nor do you. But I'll say it once more: should you ever find yourself cold, lost, alone and in genuine need of a friend... I will try to be there for you. Even if it ends up hurting me.

*What kept tipping me over subconsciously (and what must've also baffled those other guys) was the fact that we've always discussed **topics I wouldn't normally touch with a ten-foot pole** with my other female friends... and these topics were recurring themes in our conversations!*

*Our connection hasn't spiralled like this because you were 'too nice', nor is that an issue you should work on. We've ended up here because **you kept crossing boundaries**. Agreeing throughout our chats that there's mutual attraction, voicing your concerns about your past relationship patterns, hinting at asking me to help you solve your problems once and for all... Us planning exciting things to do together, talking repeatedly about sex – you hinting at it, teasing about it, telling me all the things you'd show me... whispers in doorways, wedding rings caresses, and on and on. The male brain picks up on it, and alarm bells start going off.*

According to my criteria, that's not friendship, but rather, a potential partner hinting at getting together, or at least at having affair. If you disagree with me – as I guess you will – then go on and should show your SO our chat history. I wonder how he'd judge it.

*But of course, it goes without saying that I'm equally to blame. These feelings have messed with my head – **put me in a totally different 'mode'**. When our contact oscillates wildly between maximal intimacy and 'regular friendship', my subconscious mind can't take it. Well, I guess I'm only relaxed when it comes to low stakes games. You can blame me if you so wish.*

But, I am very goal-driven by nature. Remember how I've always pushed myself, and you, to focus on our dreams? It's a boon in my life, that proclivity of mine... something I really treasure. So, I'm highly receptive to things that allow me to channel it – to people who I feel I can 'fly' towards perfection with. When you repeatedly waved that flag at me and hinted at strong interest, something deeply ingrained in me was triggered. Helping you became my mission, and I went at it in earnest. Thought I was guiding us towards a common future.

Maybe I do also have a big ego, but I guess one doesn't have to rule out the other. So, go easy on the little insults. They define you at least as much as they do me. And... they're labels too. I haven't imposed many labels on you, and did my best to shut up when you started to do things that clashed with my worldview and morals. But, I'll leave it there.

I'll keep WhatsApp downloaded. If you want to say anything else (or should you need me later to the extent that it surpasses your frustration with me), I'll be sure to reply.

I just want you to comprehend that I've finally assimilated everything and seen the connection for what it is – for what we are. I've lost you, but I've gained peace of mind. I wish you well in life.

And like that, I lost a friend, a partner in crime, a crazy, fierce, nihilist redhead, and a potential mistress who wanted to show me things I had never seen before, from my life. And, I still ached. Still couldn't sleep. Ever frantic, I looked further... dug deeper. Read about friendships, relationships, affairs. Until one day I found a term I never heard before. ...'limerent'?... Looked into it online.

That was the true missing piece of the puzzle. At last, everything fell into place and my world made sense again. Because **I fundamentally disagree with a label-less existence**. For me, knowing that others had dealt with the exact same heights of pain – and that they could be described as a tangible 'thing' – granted me my first taste of relief in months. The screaming in my head subsided, because I could point to the problem and look at it from multiple angles. My feelings weren't, in actual fact, *unique*, nor was this about 'the wonderful things' my FLO had said, or our 'special connection'.

This type of love is something else – an issue, and one that we can rip apart and understand. Can cure. A state that can be overcome, and must be overcome, by anyone prone to it. I felt compelled to re-open our WhatsApp conversation and type one last message.

*Want to know why I acted the way I did? Why you see this pattern with the guys you bond with? This missing piece, well, it's a label, but it fits. Apparently, **the cycle's called limerence**. It's what kept me up at nights, first with excitement to be with you, then in agony when I knew I never really would be.*

This particular link I'm sending you hits the nail on the head, also explaining why this is a recurring disaster for you. I know it's probably impertinent of me, but it may really help you. The good thing is, it's not truly your fault – the limerent person is always of a certain disposition, too. Obsessional, focus-oriented, etc. Bad thing is, though, there's probably a lot of homework for everyone involved.

Do with this information as you see fit. Also, check out forum posts from other limerents; 'feisty, vulnerable redhead' is clearly a recurring theme.

If this all resonates with you, please dig deeper and come to your own conclusions. This well may be the only thing of real value I ever give you. Should we ever meet again, I hope to toast to kicking Limerence. It's a monster that killed a friendship that I valued dearly.

Once you read up on this psychological state of affairs, you'll know why I must (don't want to, but must!) now uninstall WhatsApp.

Take care, redhead.

I'm not sure if she'll ever read it. But at least I tried. At least I can look at myself in the mirror again.

I tried to give her everything I had – to realign her back onto her own path. I truly tried to be there for her, and to at least *point at* what I believe to be her most destructive shortcomings. What she does with that, well, that's on her. She never owed me anything, nor I her.

Goodness, this episode cost me dearly. But I'm getting better, in all senses of the word. I realised what I really needed to do was change the way I view my FLO, as well as a tonne of psychological self-work on my own self-concept and belief systems, of course. I've ordered books on all of the new topics that I've stumbled upon over the past few months. I now feel energised and able to assess this sequence of events completely objectively, because I'm no longer running away from the truth.

I'm still healing. I still occasionally feel rough, but I'm no longer 'sick' or delusional… no longer angry. I know I'm worth it. And that my SO and our beautiful children are, too. Still, I'll be gentle with myself.

And right now, I'm mostly just trying to transform my thinking. I'm succeeding in dwelling in the correct headspace, in **embodying the correct state**. "I'm more and more at peace with my life. I'm at rest, enjoying my SO's presence and love. Here, I can breathe."

Of course, I do occasionally find myself dipping a little. Remember, limerents, the odd little tearful slump is normal during recovery. You just need your general trajectory to be moving towards emotional freedom. Want that for yourself badly enough and identify with it, and **your subconscious mind will move you towards it** – you'll heal and exit this limerence-specific feeling you're currently so caught up in.

You know, I'm actually tearing up as I write this now. But having a clear, objective understanding of what inspired my FLO to act as she did, what happened between us, **the variable rewards** and their effects on me, the shattering impact it had on my brain's biochemistry … has rescued me from the real agony that I felt only weeks ago – that I believed I'd never escape from.

It was all a fantasy. I mean, I'm so incredibly unfit to have a mistress, and that was the only type of connection that was ever possible between us. It would break my heart, and surely drive me back into the pits of the abyss. And, let's not forget that my FLO was awful for me – my connection with her left me petulant, wounded and angry. It made me act much more negatively towards my SO than she ever deserved. But, I guess little more can be expected from **a dopamine junkie in the grips of active addiction**.

I scheduled a one-on-one talk with our therapist. Asked her in advance if she had ever heard of limerence, because if not, I really wouldn't know where to start. Afterwards, I'll share the above story with my SO, to the extent that she wants to know.

Despite the above, I do strongly believe in openness in a relationship. How far I've strayed from my values, goodness... how much of a trip this has been. How good it feels to finally come back to my own essence – to my own playful way of viewing the world, and my abundance mentality. To knowing that I, and I alone, am responsible for providing myself with special, novel, exciting emotions and highs. That they're *always* within my reach... that external things are to be enjoyed and even embraced, but that assigning potent feelings to ONE fixed person/thing/place is not only unwise, but also completely *unnecessary*.

I'm Chris. And I have suffered from limerence for the last seven years. It's been nine days since I last interacted with my LO. But now? Now, I'm recovering, and I'm myself again.

All human beings are antifragile, but we limerents... even more so. Accept your feelings, analyse them, implement the correct psychological techniques and shift focus. Just **commit to getting unstuck** and to becoming a new version of yourself, and you'll be guided back towards the dance of life. And, please don't beat yourself up – chaos happens. It's about emerging stronger, and with a smile. ☺

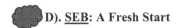 **D). <u>SEB</u>: A Fresh Start**

I've decided to share my story because I like to think it'll give future readers some hope.

I spent fifteen years of my life as a serial limerent; it all started during my teenage years, when I realised that I was gay. At the time, I wasn't accepting of my own orientation, so it goes without saying that all topics related to love were *painful* for me by default. Determined to keep my true identity a secret and 'deal with it' at some point in the future, I tried my best to focus on my work and friends – to be a 'normal teenager', just one who didn't focus on romance.

It was when I was sixteen that things started to change. I had recently started drinking and partying, and adored the new, exciting emotional intensity and opportunities for connection that exploring that side of life granted me with.

My friendship group was also perfect – I remember wishing I could freeze time, thinking "I'll never people like them again". Of course, that was (fortunately) wildly inaccurate, but that's how these things feel when you're a teenager: incredibly impactful and rare. Our nights out were magnificent, and so were our daytime adventures. Looking back, I was foolish not to come out to that group of people, as none of them would have judged me. But I just wasn't ready.

Naturally, living a lie left me very psychologically imbalanced. Craving connection and openness on a subconscious level, I was highly susceptible to 'obsessing' over anyone who **seemed to be able to read me** better than the others. Many of these obsessions were platonic, with the subjects being glamorous, popular straight girls who were particularly nice to me (in hindsight, I'm certain they sensed that I was gay). They felt like cool, accepting older sisters, and I'd think about them all the time. I had several friendships like this with girls, but there were a couple who really stood out to me as people I wanted to 'impress' – whose acceptance I craved.

Whenever I felt that my connections with one of these girls was 'deepening' (if she shared some personal information with me, complained to me about her boyfriend, or took a photo with me), I'd be left euphoric. Since the bulk of my life involved me living very inauthentically, these little moments of intimacy hit me so, so hard. All I wanted was to 'know' that I was *always* going to be supported, encouraged and accepted by these girls. That they were always going to want to tell me their secrets. Crazy as it sounds, nothing would have delighted me more than if one of them had written me a formal letter promising to 'be my friend forever'. I felt like I needed a *guarantee* that they **wouldn't grow bored of me**.

I now find it fascinating to reflect on this adolescent tendency of mine to 'bond' with strong, popular girls who showed me affection– despite it being **completely platonic obsession**, it was the first instance of **my limerent disposition** cropping up. It indicated that I had enough psychological issues to be *able* to fixate on a person (and what they could offer me emotionally) in the first place, and *subsequently* find my mood controlled by them. By how interested I believed them to be in the connection advancing.

So, it isn't surprising that I eventually fell into **real, romantic limerence**. I fell head-over-heels 'in love' with my straight best friend two months before I turned seventeen. The classic coming-of-age story, and an insufferable trope, I know. But it really happened to me. What had started out as a really **interesting, enlivening friendship**, involving us partying, riding our bikes together and looking for animals in the forest, turned into me craving his attention every waking moment of my life.

I think all limerents can relate to what you astutely describe as 'limerence crystallisation' – when you look at your LO, and you realise "oh dear... I don't just feel happy in this person's presence. I'm absolutely obsessed with them; they're pure magic". One morning, we were lazily riding our bikes along our favourite canal, and I felt it incredibly strongly for the first time – that special 'him' feeling. Realised that it was there to stay, and that I was going to suffer from it, badly. That something about it was too real. This was something I had never felt for anyone before, as my earlier crushes had been fairly ephemeral – I hadn't shared intense emotional connections with them, or admired them. I hadn't found myself giddy with joy or petrified.

Given my inability to disclose my feelings, I suffered in silence, braving my way through each school day but breaking down in tears every night. As is the case with **any form of first love** (whether normal or limerent), this boy had a ridiculously strong influence on me in general. I emulated so many things about him, because he inspired me. Found myself going on more bike rides, and getting into nature photography – two of his favourite hobbies. Also read a lot of magical realism books, because he was an avid fan of Murakami. To be honest, reading those highly evocative novels only worsened my state because I felt that I identified with many of the protagonists: guys who pined from a distance, but couldn't quite express their feelings…or knew that doing so would be in vain. Flies on the wall, wasted love, etc. I found *Norwegian Wood* particularly devastating.

I pined like this for <u>two whole years</u>, never once daring to have a sincere conversation with him about how I felt. And gosh, how that limerent episode coloured that period of my youth and distinguished it from the rest of my adolescence, which I now remember as light, playful and manageable in comparison. There had been brutal lows, I'm sure, but nothing like those that my first limerent episode subjected me to.

When I went to university to study business, **I fell for another guy**: my heterosexual flatmate. My feelings for my first LO rapidly faded, and we also drifted as friends as a result – there was no longer anything intense binding us together. We had become so close in the first place because I had been *obsessively infatuated with him*. Despite being quite good at hiding my feelings, I had prioritised him above everything else and always proactively helped him resolve any issues that came his way. And he, as a result, had grown to care for me in an incredibly deep (albeit entirely platonic) way. But, our shared 'magic' simply vanished when I no longer saw him through the **delusory, distorted goggles** of limerence.

Our paths sharply bifurcated, and the strangest thing was, I didn't even care. Nothing about him really stood out to me or resonated with me anymore. It was like those feelings had just been *transferred* to my new LO, with whom I lived and shared a lot of formative university experiences. Honestly, there's no point me elaborating much on this second limerent episode, because it mimicked my first one, uncannily. At the time, I failed to see this, because limerence always tells you that 'this time it's rational/real love/not an illusion', and also that your current LO (and what s/he stirs up in you) has 'nothing to do with your previous LOs'. But, limerence is always about you, and there's always a clear pattern going on behind the scenes… behind the madness.

I can speak for myself and say that both my first and second limerent episodes were predominantly defined by my desire to bond with a **confident, extroverted guy**, **be wholly understood by him** and *feel free/powerful*. By completely ignoring my own psychological needs and failing to be brave and honest about my orientation, I was allowing myself to attract limerence, and nothing more than limerence. My 'trigger archetype' was very specific, but equally could have been fulfilled by a lot of guys (probably why I'm a serial limerent). They just had to be warm (at least initially), more adventurous than me, open-minded enough to entertain a deep, intimate 'friendship' (I only fell for guys who spent a lot of time with me), but who kept me at a distance and were occasionally a little cold (that essential intermittent reward).

Needless to say, this pattern continued unfolding in my life. I won't describe the *subsequent* two limerent episodes (LE3 and LE4!) I fell into during my twenties, because they were both very similar to the first two. Savage, devastating, derailing and humiliating. They truly did a number on my mental health, and my work and friendships suffered massively. I did want to recover and approach romance normally, but my feelings stopped me advancing because **I bought into them far too much**. Each time I was limerent, I'd swear that 'this time it's different. I'm not sick, I'm in love. And, I can't let this person go.'

Oh, and these two LOs were also straight men. Since I was living life as someone who 'would never be authentic or live out a real relationship', I had limited my *actual* connections with men to casual dating. I specifically targeted out individuals I could be somewhat attracted to but who I knew *I'd never fall for*. Who were as committed to 'not catching feelings' for anyone as I was. I definitely have the obsessive-leaning limerent mentality by nature, but by living like this, I was unknowingly **creating a space in my life for limerence**. And, in turn, *denying myself* the chance of experiencing real romance.

I was unknowingly sending my own subconscious mind a clear message: that I didn't want to be **pushed into 'that corner'** – into a real, requited relationship with feelings, that would force me to come out of the closet and display *my whole truth* to the world. And, it complied with my request to a T, encouraging me to become smitten with straight guys who were absolutely off the cards from the get-go.

Luckily, there's a happy ending here. I eventually made peace with myself and my identity, and have cured myself of this nightmare. My final (and fifth) limerent episode struck me at the end of my twenties, but it was slightly different to those that preceded it; my LO was, for the first time, another gay man. I had recently decided to take the plunge and rip off the plaster – to dare myself to **start dating guys seriously**, in the hope of finding a stable, enriching romantic relationship.

Sick of limiting myself to painful, unrequited feelings for unattainable straight guys, I simply decided to have faith, and to believe in my ability to attract something I had *never quite seen* materialise in my reality before. I decided to trust in the overarching mantra preached by most branches of spirituality: that changing your 'inner world' will always impact your outer reality. That you're always better off focusing on a new, desirable outcomes than 'logically' reflecting on how badly things have previously gone for you. Because doing so will only ever bring you more of the same.

I now know that mantra to be one hundred percent true. Turns out, when I first approached dating guys in a more emotional way, I was still carrying around a lot of baggage. My 'trigger archetype' had changed from 'heterosexual guy who can provide me with *some* emotional intimacy' to 'authentic gay guy who'll help me through this transition phase'.

My fifth LO certainly did serve this purpose, and I will forever be grateful for having met him; he was uninhibited, crazy and carefree. However, he was also **a nasty piece of work**, subjecting me to gaslighting, chaos and misery. Out of the five LOs I've had throughout my lifetime, he was the only one who I can genuinely say had terrible, twisted intentions; the rest were, of course, just straight guys who didn't want to date me. But who, by being extremely open (and not maintaining conventional, rigid boundaries that straight guys typically uphold with other men), provided me with scraps of what I wanted at the time: connection.

In contrast, my final limerent episode came along with some severe, real-life ramifications. This guy stole from me (despite me always lending him what he needed to fund his lavish, outlandish lifestyle), and invented stories about me. Tried to claim to *my own friends* that I'd done heinous things, and that *he* was the victim in the relationship. He was trouble from the get-go; now, I'd know to immediately nip a similar connection in the bud, because I'd see *nothing special or interesting* in that level of craziness. Nothing mysterious or quirky. But I was vulnerable at the time, and felt that I couldn't quite live as an 'out' gay man without his help – without his bold, 'who cares what they think anyway?' demeanour.

Thankfully, I **discovered the term 'limerence'** five months after we officially separated and cut contact (during which time I thought about him and mourned his energy in my life *relentlessly*).

Educating myself on this condition, and the real, tangible psychological and neuroscientific basis of it all, saved my life. That I can say without hesitation. I couldn't be more grateful to have discovered this book (and your content), in particular. I've since completely reprogrammed my subconscious mind, healed my wounds, and stepped into a completely new identity. It sounds crazy, but I often catch myself **thinking, feeling a specific way, or acting,** and realise that I would have never done so six months ago – that I would've responded differently to that particular situation, or ended up feeling differently and spiralling into negativity.

Most importantly, I know myself to now be 'limerence immune'. As someone who works in a large, progressive company, I come across countless bright, warm, intelligent people who I realise have *many of the traits* that affected me so obsessively ***to the point of addiction*** in the past. The traits that once sent me spiralling into limerence for months or years, all because my own psychological issues let them do so. To realise that the very people who would've sent you off the rails emotionally in the past now **barely even catch your attention** is just incredible.

I won't say the obvious, because you readers all know what you need to do now: commit to overcoming this madness, treat yourself with self-love, integrate all aspects of your nature/personality, and above all, view life *playfully*. Nothing's fixed or that serious – you can always get yourself on a new path, regardless of where you currently are. But, you must trust in your ability to change… and in the ability of your reality to mirror this change.

There is one particularly priceless lesson that limerence has taught me. One that I'd like to leave you readers with. It's that you must be very, very careful which conversations you have with yourself. Your thoughts (and internal narratives) really do create your reality, because they establish your intentions – and your brain will always force you to act/feel/think in a way that **fulfils your innermost intentions**. Identify them and change those that are problematic, or your brain will constantly generate emotions that will drive you towards responses and actions that keep you trapped in a life you don't want. Emotions that will ultimately sabotage you.

As someone who disliked biology in school, I never envisaged that I'd find myself interested in neuroscience in my early thirties. But overcoming limerence and transforming more than I ever thought was possible has left me insatiably curious about the innermost workings of the brain. It's the most marvellous computer out there, but it's ultimately just designed to do its job – **to edge you closer to goals** that you've set for yourself (whether consciously or not), by controlling how you act.

And how does it control how you act? It achieves this by eliciting specific emotional responses in you – for example, in limerence, it allows LOs of a specific nature to make you euphoric, driving you to do embarrassing things to 'get closer' to them.

Luckily, you can radically alter your intentions through subconscious mind reprogramming (particularly through hypnosis and affirmations that *stir up different emotions*). This is the foundation of any type of psychological transformation, but is particularly powerful when it comes to limerence, romance, etc. You'll see how quickly you grow tired of chasing after your LO – how their lustre starts to fade, and they impact you less and less. Other people's reactions to you will also change, and in turn, you'll attract new experiences, opportunities, conversations and connections almost like magic.

NOTE FROM THE AUTHOR: this individual has hit the nail on the head; your brain will always influence you to act in such a way that your deeply rooted goals/intentions are fulfilled. This is one of the predominant things that separates people who achieve amazing things 'ease', and those who 'lack discipline'. The subconscious minds of the former are *working in coherence* with their conscious interests/desires. The result is that they're 'impulsed' to do the right things, and act in such a way that they will be brought closer to what they want. Even though they will, of course, still struggle with aspects of life and occasionally cycle through negative emotions, they'll be acting beneficially to their interests most of the time. This is because their brains will be generating the correct emotions, which will elicit the correct actions/behaviour from them fairly automatically.

The nature of your goal/intention does not matter: whether you want to get fit, feel more focused during the day, earn a certain amount per month from an online business or attract a very specific, requited relationship dynamic, you must **ensure that you truly want** all of what will come with the 'prize'. And if you do, employ visualisation techniques etc. to drive this message home to your subconscious mind – **think from the end**.

However, I must clarify one thing. This individual is absolutely correct in implying that setting intentions is an essential part of limerence recovery (and success in all domains of life). This is, after all, what much of the subconscious mind programming detailed in this book achieves → it launches you towards a new self-concept that encapsulates new interests/dreams/desires/goals. But, don't forget how important it is that you **first identify/correct your unmet needs**. i.e. what is it about your LO in particular that makes you feel so 'high'?

Because, as we've covered, a bad limerent episode always follows an initial 'glimmer' – the initial dopamine saturation that you receive from noticing that something about your LO makes you feel better/safe/liberated/just amazing. The goal in recovery is to re-build yourself into a version of yourself who wouldn't be able to feel that same 'glimmer', should you meet your LO again. Who may feel some attraction, admiration or interest, but all within the 'normal, manageable human range'; a version of yourself who would never, ever be able to entertain the idea of throwing away your life for this person.

Sometimes our tendency **to fall for a particular type of person** *disappear*s when we reshuffle our priorities, belief systems and intentions/goals. For example, the author of this previous account found that his desire to 'enmesh' with straight men who couldn't ever reciprocate his feelings vanished when he <u>worked on establishing new beliefs</u> regarding his worth/ability to live openly and honestly. The fact that his subsequent LO was an gay man who happened to be a little unstable *perfectly* reflected his changed beliefs and intentions ('I can go beyond casual dating and find a requited emotional connection with another man' but 'I want to attract someone intense, because I don't yet feel fully authentic myself'). In this way, he overcame his tendency to fall for his previous trigger archetype (straight guy, warm but a little distant...) the second he modified his beliefs and intentions. When he dared to 'push' his brain into 'seek emotional connection with someone who can reciprocate' mode, he fell limerent for a guy who he did, at least, date for a while.

However, altering your intentions can only go so far when you're limerence-prone. There will always be unmet needs beneath the surface, and they'll will crop up in different ways until you deal with them. Sometimes they are circumstantial (this individual, for example, desperately needed to start living authentically to *permanently overcome limerence* – to do himself justice by accepting himself wholeheartedly). This does not mean that such unmet needs don't run deep and cause trouble in many facets of your life, for most certainly do. It just means that they are easily resolved by making one (often not easy) <u>decision</u>.

Most of the time, however, unmet needs are **more reflective of your general nature** than any one decision that you have made in life. For example, if you're starting to gather that you need to become more spontaneous, expressive and bold (because your LOs have always been unstable, borderline personality disorder-leaning individuals), you can consider this a more 'general' unmet need. One that requires **<u>intervention on many different levels</u>**. To free yourself from limerence, you'll need to prioritise new, fun feelings in your life and opportunities for you to enter special 'flow states' (with people and in your work/hobbies) that connect you with your heart. Only then will you be *immune to* potential future LOs who flash you that 'authenticity glimmer' that has previously got you so hooked. Only then will these characters take on normal, human qualities, allowing you to deal with them without being triggered in the slightest.

So, **the upshot here** is that you must consider whether your unmet needs have arisen because of one clear lifestyle choice (that you can rapidly alter, even if doing so is out of your comfort zone), OR whether they are the cumulative result of years of living slightly in fear/*against your nature/accepting dullness*. If the former, you must take the plunge and change that one thing in your life; this may well be sufficient to immunise you against limerence. However, if the latter, you must commit to engaging in lots of different activities, meeting new people and *thinking* in completely refreshed ways in order to live in consonance with **your intrinsic needs**.

Once you're getting to grips with handing your psychological needs in this way (i.e. distinguishing between which are relatively general/reflective of your intrinsic nature, and which are 'created' (whether through specific lifestyle choices OR past influences beyond your control)), the subconscious mind reprogramming techniques we have already covered will be immensely powerful.

This is because when your needs are no longer chronically unmet, you will **no longer feel terrible**. Consequently, you will also no longer be operating in a scarcity mentality or 'blocking' yourself from reaching higher states of consciousness. In this vastly ameliorated psychological state, your subconscious mind will be highly receptive to your active efforts to imprint it with new, positive ideas and beliefs. You will be well-poised to see magical results in your life from merely **setting new intentions** through goal-focused subconscious programming (visualising, thinking from the end etc.); it will work seamlessly. You'll be in charge of your 'computer' of a brain *once and for all*, and will be able to align with the specific **limerence-immune self-concept** AND lifestyle that you desire. Down to the very last detail.

If you try to establish new intentions/alter your self-concept in this way *before* you start to deal with your unmet needs, however, you may struggle. This is because you will still be dealing with *the most severe* of your limerent lows, rendering imprinting your brain with the idea of pleasant, exciting things as easy as *baptising a cat*. It's possible to transform your intentions/self-concept from this place of chaos and agony, but measurably more difficult. It is for this reason that it is paramount that you view limerence *in terms of your psychological needs* before anything else. In terms of what you feel that your LO provides you with (whether something very clear and obvious such as physical protection, or something subtle like the authenticity they radiate through their 'quirky' messaging style).

Once you understand your limerence pattern from this angle (i.e. *what are my unmet needs?*), you will possess incredible leverage and the subconscious mind techniques <u>will work very rapidly for you</u>. You'll start to see the fruits of your labour reflected in your thoughts, feelings, attitude and your behaviour (i.e. what situations/conversations you naturally fall into) in a matter of days. Seeing these changes will be extremely exciting for you, and unlike anything you have ever experienced before – remember, most people never learn how to **speak to their subconscious minds** and elicit crazy, magnificent changes in their lives. Most people believe that their inner states, feelings about themselves/others and actions are somewhat 'fixed'.

From this point onwards, you'll be able to continue with the techniques and see through your entire **recovery from limerence** with ease and optimism.

 E). <u>MARIA</u>: Long Distance, Emotional Distance Or Both?

Here's my story. Interestingly, after this last episode hit me, I realised that I've probably been or in and out of limerence my entire adult life. It's hard to tell now. I dealt with this extreme limerent episode last year; it started in June and 'ended' in December. He's come back into my field of vision, and I'm still fearful of falling back into the same state. But, I do feel much stronger at this point.

I met him on eHarmony on the 5th of May. He's from Colorado and I live in New Jersey – I had previously widened my search parameters to include places I'd consider moving to. We texted for a week or two, and the interest seemed mutual. We made plans to meet on the 24th of June, and he flew me out there using his miles for a long weekend. However, we only spoke around four times between matching online and me visiting him (red flag!).

When we met in person, I liked him immediately and he liked me too. We hiked, walked around town, and much to my surprise, I ended up being intimate with him that weekend. I never thought that would happen......and it was great. I'm not used to it being great, to say the least. But on the way to the airport before I even flew home, something was said and I felt some emotional distance between us......and his response was "here we go." HUGE red flag. Dismissive – insulting even. I left his state, just like that – felt hugely dejected.

In the ensuing two months, over which time he had made plans to visit me in NJ, I spoke to him about once a week. I decided to be explicit and tell him that **once a week is not enough** to keep a long distance relationship going. He is **anathema to the word relationship** and responded reluctantly: "can't we just let things develop naturally?"

Although I hardly knew this guy, and it was becoming increasingly evident that he was not emotionally available, I found myself obsessed with him, waiting on his texts (and calls, which rarely came). I even realised that this was probably his 'style.' He had been married for twenty-five years, but admittedly, had only ever been at home for around 20% of the time due to being a submariner. After that marriage, he dated a different woman for seven years – they had just broken up when we connected. He also told me he travelled much of that time. This was clearly a man who was used to not connecting.....but, I still believed that things could, and would, change.

In reality, his visit to NJ was not great... except for the sex. He was distracted with work stuff, cheap with meals, off during conversations. When he left, I drove him an hour and a half to the airport but decided against putting myself through the overnight wait with him for his early trip, instead going home. I KNEW that it wasn't working, that the connection wasn't blossoming as it should. But nonetheless, I tried to persuade him to make a deal to call me three times a week. Before December came around, he showed me that he wasn't capable of that (said he didn't like being told what he was supposed to do). **He ghosted me at the end of December**.

He *has* texted me since then. I'd deleted his phone number, so had to ask who it was. I don't feel the same way, which is a huge relief! **I'm no longer limerent** – no longer craving the scraps of attention that he'd throw me without showing any signs of wanting to emotionally invest.

I could embellish this story with many more details, but I wanted to keep it simple. I like to think it'll help people see the true nature of what this madness is – transient emotions, and nothing more. Something that you can, and will, recover from. But, the root causes must be addressed and treated, or you'll fall for the next person who resembles your current LO.

Oddly, I'd had a book on limerence on my bookshelf for years, and didn't even really know what it was about. Read it in Sept/Oct and wow.....what a revelation.

Thank you for your work. I just went to visit another potential guy in a different state, and the same thing almost happened. I read your book in one sitting that day... another long story. But, doing so completely prevented me from falling down the same rabbit hole – completely enabled me to see the connection for what it was, and laugh at the idea of someone *taking on that much meaning* in my head.

Romance isn't meant to be so colossal, so damaging. Keep it simple, sweet and real, because when it's real, it is simple and sweet... and enjoy life. Be aware of the beauty that surrounds you, and access highs and good feelings in as many *healthy* ways as you possibly can.

F). <u>ABIONA</u>: Multiple LOs, Multiple Worlds

I can't believe I'm at a point where I feel completely safe from the grips of limerence – completely recovered and lucid. That I was actually able to respond to your website post asking for us to share our stories. Three months ago, I wouldn't have been *able* to sit down and write about my experience … It would've triggered me and made me tearful, maybe even pushing me into a slump and threatening my productivity for days.

I lived walking on eggshells, but I'm now free – free to feel and free to live, rid of the parasite that is pathological, delusional love. I owe virtually all of my current mental stability and peace of mind to *this very book*, so it's exciting to know that my story will be included in the updated version. Sharing it is the least I can do. I like to think that future readers will be able to relate to some of the specific feelings I try (potentially in vain!) to describe. Or that hearing my story might draw their attention to elements of their own experiences that they hadn't placed much importance on before.

I'm in my mid-twenties and am halfway through **my PhD in Chemistry**. I've always greatly enjoyed the subject and had an analytical mind, whilst also loving films, books, music and the rest. The classic limerent disposition, or so it seems... enough obsessional focus to really fixate on a goal, but enough of a lover of spontaneity/life to allow love (albeit delusional love) to actually *become* one of my big goals. I've come to see that not everyone who's prone to systemising and overthinking will ever experience limerence, nor will everyone who's passionate and interested in people. Your disposition needs to be a mix of those two extremes, or to at least be capable of channelling a mix of them at certain times.

But, enough abstractions. I'll dive right into my story.

I'm prone to incredibly strong feelings in general, but what I've felt for the two LOs I've had in my life has been **ridiculously, sickeningly strong**. As will be the case for every limerent who ever tries to articulate anything about the state, I'm frustrated as I type – language is so limited. Even the most emphatic words probably only describe around 30% of the pain, and the euphoria, that limerence has subjected me to. It's truly something else.

I experienced crushes as a teenager, which were definite obsessions but nothing that ever developed into full-blown limerence. I thought a lot about those individuals (girls and boys, as I'm bisexual) and stalked them incessantly on social media, but the feelings never seemed capable of making me depressed. I never felt like my entire reward system was awaiting their attention – was never stuck by that **horrible, quintessentially 'limerent' feeling** that has you sitting alone in your room in the deepest depths of despair, feeling like you'll <u>never see value in anyone or anything</u> that isn't your LO. Goodness, what a delusion the whole condition is. How amazing it is to be over it.

Recent introspection has lead me to see why I never fell into true 'limerence' for these people at school, despite obviously being genetically wired for the condition. As a teenager, I was introverted, awkward and terrified of the popular kids. I didn't express who I was or even *know* who I was/what I liked; my personality simply wasn't developed enough for me to have

a magical mental 'click' with anyone. You see, your writing has taught me so many fascinating things – above all, it's really woken me up to the fact that the neural makeup you're born with determines whether you *could* one day become limerent, but ***precise psychological factors*** actually determine *whether you'll experience it*. For you to experience limerence (i.e. spot the glimmer in someone and subsequently fall into addiction), you need to have unmet psychological needs and be in a particular headspace.

Curiously, I'm most vulnerable to limerence when I'm in love with what I'm doing, inspired by others around me (and generally receptive to people), but somehow **convinced that my life could be even more blissful** if I had access to *different* 'energy'. Energy that my life isn't quite providing me with. It's ONLY in this state that I'm able to lock eyes with someone and see so much potential in them –potential to make my life a wonderful, colourised dream.

You see, at school, I was on autopilot and lived in fear. Sure, there were happy moments, but I wasn't subconsciously looking for life to feel like a dream. I didn't know that it could feel like a dream. So, despite being unhappier and less well-rounded than I am now, I was strangely safe from limerence as a teenager. I didn't project that 'unmet need'/desire onto anyone, because I didn't have that much poetic 'intensity' inside myself back then. I was able to just develop normal crushes for the special people I did encounter, and always got over them three months later.

LOs have to represent a tonne to you, on a spiritual and emotional level, to drive you so crazy. I wasn't aligned or mentally stimulated enough in life for my brain to undergo that **initial dopamine flood**… for it to start to associate *anything or anyone* with the idea of true bliss. I guess I was just in survival mode. I wasn't tapping into my goal-setting side, which meant I wasn't capable of entertaining *any* big goals – limerence, of course, is the ultimate form of goal-seeking behaviour… just channelled towards romance (much to our detriment).

But that soon changed – when I got to university, a whole new world opened up for me. I adored my subject and became highly perfectionistic, driven to score as highly as I could in every single exam. Getting those grades felt glorious, simply wonderful – I had performed well in school because I naturally excelled at maths and the sciences, but I never really felt like my success was intentional. I believe that your **success must be conscious**, or you will always suffer your successes. They'll feel a little like gambling, like you don't quite deserve the prize. You'll be scared of losing it, and often will lose it.

Well, at university, everything about my life became conscious. I tabulated my academic progress, branched out socially, and also threw myself into running and strength training. However cheesy it may sound, I felt *in love with life* for the first time. I realised that I could actually carve out my own destiny, and started to see everything like a game – my quest was to level up in as many areas as possible. I also exuded a certain magnetic quality that I hadn't before. I knew that people were perceiving the real me – they didn't always like me, but people never forgot me, because I was a lot more 'awake' than the average person.

Of course, I attribute this entirely to my mentality shift, and some techniques I'd implement. Every hour, I'd make a habit of grounding myself and thinking "who am I? Where am I? What am I doing right now", which I highly recommend that everyone reading this tries. My mentality was more sharp, focused and positive than ever as a result. I aligned with some really magical friends around that time, who I'm still incredibly close with to this day.

Being more 'awake' also gave me the newfound ability to click with people I was *truly* romantically interested in: **highly perfectionistic, driven, passionate** people. Previously, I bizarrely hadn't really noticed such individuals, and they hadn't noticed or felt drawn to me, either. But, it was like we were suddenly resonating at the same frequency and *a match*. One of them I dated for a year – a lovely guy who I ended up breaking up with because the relationship was too time-consuming. I initially loved him, but that love evolved into something more complacent and capable of resentment. I wanted to be my ambitious, 'solo warrior' self again, disliking how content and relaxed I had become during our relationship.

It wasn't like this guy actively hindered my progress, but he just didn't share my drive for growth and improvement. This lead to me constantly feeling like I was *dragging him along with me* while he just about complied – a feeling I despised. I wanted someone who would *pull ME along* even higher than I'd naturally dare to go myself: the opposite of him. That was my fantasy... something I felt I really needed in a partner.

In hindsight, this 'unmet need' of mine was precisely what set me up for falling for my first LO, who I met at the beginning of my final undergraduate year. I now know that I didn't really *need* someone to be more 'focused/ambitious' than me – I needed to learn to tune into my softer sides and reward myself when I actually hit my goals. Have more compassion for myself, and stop pushing myself so hard; to practise self-directed gratitude, and celebrate my little wins *myself*. **Taking care of myself like that was my *true* unmet need**, little did I know. But, back to my first LO, and what I perceived that he provided me with.

I first spoke to him in labs, and immediately felt drawn to him. He was tall and slightly lanky, with piercing blue eyes and light brown hair. Had a lively regional accent, as he was from our university city. We made small talk about the work we were doing, but I could tell what it all meant to him, there and then in the fluorescently lit lab – his eyes sparkled and he just radiated energy, as he smirked at me. I instantly knew that university life meant a tonne to him, too. That he'd recently learnt to tap into his true intellectual capabilities and was consciously creating his life like I was, incredibly excited about the future. That he was also capable of that **goal-oriented euphoria** that I knew so well and loved so much... and that he similarly prioritised dipping into it every day, actively rejecting safe, cosy, mundane things.

With his unique *joie de vivre*, he was <u>unlike anyone else</u> I knew at the time – a league above them all. What luck, finding him.

Most students our age bonded over what was 'relatable': complaining, talking negatively about the future, sharing insecurities etc. But, like me, he didn't want to hear any of it – such limiting self-talk simply didn't exist in his reality. He was kind to everyone and would help anyone who was struggling, but he wasn't going to assimilate one fragment of their limiting, negative energy. He wasn't narcissistic at all, but rather, a dreamer who was committed to *also* being a go-getter. He trusted in his ability to secure whatever he wanted in life and access whatever emotions he wanted, but there was no arrogance in the mix – he came across as polite, warm and unassuming. He just seemed 'awake', and was the only 'awake' person my age that I'd spoken to in weeks. He was strong, cheery, completely void of any pettiness and incapable of complaining, because he saw an amazing future laid out for him that just required him to 'play the part'.

This **beautiful, clean stoicism** that he effortlessly channelled made me feel wonderful. It made me think of sunlight, mountains and carefree, roaming animals. It sounds crazy, but he genuinely stirred up this imagery in me from the first day that we met – everyone in your life comes to represent things (platonic friends, family etc.), but this boy simply WAS these things to me: freedom, peace, security, growth. An incredibly intoxicating mix. With him, and him alone, I seemed to be guaranteed permanent access to a life boasting these sublime qualities and experiences.

Our connection blossomed in a real, requited way, and I felt protected by him – loved him. I remember waking up and thinking "**love is either a yes or a no**, and I'm obviously in love. It's as opaque and real as a brick wall, what I feel for this boy." At that time, my feelings were genuine and sustainable. He pursued me a little more than I pursued him, and it seemed to be developing into a real relationship.

He truly embodied the personality that my subconscious had been tuned to seek before we first clicked… certainly **my 'trigger archetype' at that point in my life**. Finally, I had found a partner who I felt was 'higher-value' than me in some way (I hate to use such terms, but they can be useful in this context – power dynamics do accompany limerence, which one of your online posts opened my eyes up to). Rather than me feeling like I was the achiever who had to 'drag him along' reluctantly while he supported me, I got to watch him ace life, too. I respected and adored him, thanking the universe that I had been given this opportunity to love and actually *admire* someone who was simultaneously jokey, relaxed and, of course, as young as I was.

I hated to admit it, but he also made me reflect further on my previous relationship. I could no longer deny it; there had always been something downright ingratiating about that look in my former boyfriend's eyes when I'd wanted to go out and do something… supportive, full of admiration, but somehow simultaneously imploring me to stay with him. It had *angered* me – made me yearn for **someone to sometimes leave *me* behind**, to prioritise themself. To head out, impassioned and excited to explore a facet of life that didn't involve me. I think I knew that a connection of this nature would subconsciously motivate me to be **my very best**

self at all times (productive, feminine, cheerful, physically fit, energetic, soft, loving), in order to 'keep' them.

I really just wanted to feel sky-high euphoria, and power, at that point in my life. Being that version of myself gave me access to those feelings. Finally, I had someone who incentivised me to be 'That' Me; to smash my exams, stay in shape, and also live a rich emotional life.

However, five months later, things started to go a little pear-shaped. I won't go into too much depth here, but it was like we started to snap out of the lovey-dovey 'trance' we'd been in – or, rather, we were jolted involuntarily out of the state we'd initially put each other in. As the weeks passed, I realised that **our perfect synchrony** – that delicious feeling of us both growing and smashing our goals – only existed when I was in a very particular headspace. When I was a little 'low', or complained a bit, we clashed. It was like he no longer saw that magic in me, and was disappointed... disappointed that I wasn't the Queen-like character who had initially piqued his interest in labs – the girl who was ultra-productive and determined, but also smiley, positive and playful 24/7... his dream woman.

I remember thinking "Ironically, I've got exactly what I want – someone who's more stoic than me, and better-equipped to cut through life and achieve things than me. Who's very similar to me but *not* plagued by my emotions or my weaknesses – **my stronger half, and a mentor**. Someone who I know *doesn't like or accept* every single version of me, and who is never going to be so desperate they stick around if/when I'm at my worst. Someone who, because of all of this, motivates me to be my very best self without having to say a word. But, I don't know if I can hold onto this. I feel like he's slipping through my fingers."

The issue was, I couldn't sustain that specific 'dream version of myself' with him. The irony doesn't escape me here, given that his influence in my life initially aligned me closer than ever with my best self. But, that initial honeymoon phase where your mood is *wholly and positively influenced* by the fact that you're in requited love wanes. Life got in the way, my mood dipped, work piled up, friends would bombard me with issues, and I'd slip a little in *some* regard. Slip away from that ideal. He, on the other hand, never seemed to slip; his baseline state was simply superior to mine.

It was crazy; he seemed perpetually under the influence of a hyper-masculine, stoic life force (albeit one that I had certainly never seen in any other guy) – he'd jump out of bed, never skipped a gym session, read every morning, and drifted through the campus greeting Professors and students warmly. Never a down day, never a spiralling episode leading to him doubting himself. **Nothing irrational**, nothing overly emotional. Importantly, his virtues extended far beyond his productivity – he seemed to manage to juggle everything, also staying on top of politics, and attending random casual lunches with our classmates. Many of which I would skip – all the studying and caffeine-consuming made me a little socially anxious during the day, and I didn't feel that I could just flexibly and spontaneously socialise with those smart, earnest people during the week. I needed to hype myself up beforehand.

Needless to say, we began to drift and eventually broke up. I now see that it *wasn't* the fact that I 'wasn't perfect all the time' that lead to his becoming disillusioned with me. Rather, **it was my fear of losing him** - it was the fact that I was too obsessively in love with 'him' (or, really, what he represented to me/who I thought I was, and was becoming, with him in my life). But, the brusque curtailment of our requited relationship is not the focus of this story, nor is it that big of a deal; looking back, I'm glad we didn't stay together.

What is relevant, however, is the fact that I spent the ensuing year in **absolute limerent chaos**. I couldn't get over him - couldn't deal with my emotions. Couldn't kiss goodbye to the world that he had opened up for me.

Finishing my Chemistry degree whilst dealing with crippling depression and manic highs and lows was a *suboptimal experience*, to say the least. Looking back, I am amazed I pulled through - amazed I didn't develop substance abuse issues, or drop out of university. But, I powered through, aware that I was in a delusional and transient state (for I had **started to research limerence** and found that it described my state perfectly). I eventually finished with very high grades, and was instantly accepted onto my dream PhD programme at a university in my home city. One renowned for my subject and for its progressive, liberal ethos.

On a logical level, I was delighted. I knew that I had carved out something wonderful for myself… that all my work had not been in vain. That I'd be able to call myself Dr. four years later. But I couldn't feel any joy. It was six months after our break up, and I was still stuck in that **loathsome state of lovesickness**. I'd roll my eyes at myself and think "dream big! Get excited about the future and forget him! You'll meet more stimulating people", but I didn't believe I would. Since this was my first time being limerent, I was truly stuck in the delusion that the magnitude and intensity of my feelings 'meant something of epic and colossal significance' – that I craved this guy because I HAD to have him. That I was cheating myself of a full life if I didn't get him back.

Needless to say, I still had one foot stuck in the past and was pretty much *doing the opposite* of the techniques that do, truly, let you recover. I was just about aware that I needed to get over him, but acting in a way that was ***simply not conducive*** to me achieving this. In addition to allowing myself to think/write about him on a daily basis (from the 'woe is me' victim headspace), I was allowing him to represent a tonne to me - I still subconsciously believed that I was 'at my best' with him, and that in his absence, life was always bound to be a **messy, superficial, pointless farce**. I didn't put any effort into catalysing the establishment of new belief systems within me, or even properly *counter* such thoughts.

Incidentally, my ability to be frivolous and happy for 'no reason' plummeted to zero. I'd go to my friends' parties and try and focus on how much platonic love I housed for them, telling myself that THEY were there for me, and this guy wasn't. But I'd just find myself depressed in their company, faking smiles and laughter but focusing on all of their flaws. You see, they all lacked his smart, disciplined 'poise' … his intense desire to capitalise on every twenty-four hour period he was given on this planet. They lacked his essence, which I loved and craved so much.

Because it wasn't really about intelligence. My friends were very bright in different ways, but even the most conventionally academic-leaning of them would complain about certain aspects of their university experience (which is, in reality, normal and healthy). However, compared to this guy's **compelling, admirable stoicism and focus**, it made them seem childish and *limiting* to me – one-dimensional.

"If he were here, he wouldn't judge the others for complaining, but he'd smile and put a playful, positive spin on the situation", I'd think. I hated myself for it, but I found myself resenting my friends' sloppy attitudes towards work and life, and wanting to distance myself from them. This caused me to become livid with myself – livid that I was obsessed with a guy who didn't want me (who I was convinced was 'perfect'), and even more **livid that I was turning bitter** and judging my lovely friends. Furious that shifting myself out of this state wasn't proving easy – that I was even more miserable at parties and birthday dinners than I was *when I cried, alone, in my room*.

It was a horrible time for me, full of immense self-hatred, guilt and panic. However, I did, at least, start to *seriously* accept that what I was feeling **was not meaningful love**. That it was seriously detrimental issue that I had to fight. I just didn't know how, other than to keep forcing myself to socialise with people I didn't want to see (and who just made my LO's virtues seem even more rare, and precious). If only this book had existed back then - I would've realised what I really needed to do to stop the pain was *design a new self-concept*. Fall in love with new states, plan my future PhD life, and factor in things/goals he couldn't be part of, etc. That'd have saved me in a matter of weeks.

Instead, convinced that I had to 'replace' my feelings with something else equally impactful, **I fell for someone else** – for a second LO. Yes, really; I met someone that summer, before my PhD programme started, and let them induce the same type of chaos in me that this guy had.

When you don't realise that you're the ticking time bomb, it's inevitable that you'll keep wreaking havoc. Clearly, *I had no idea* that my root issues were my unmet needs, my beliefs about myself, this guy and what was possible for me, and, by extension, how I viewed and felt about myself. I naively thought that my intense, unhealthy 'love' for him was a one-off – a logical reaction to the Perfect Guy I had met, and not *really* a reflection of my own mentality. That it 'wouldn't happen again' – limerence could be a one-time thing, right?

My second LO was a girl. I met her that summer after my undergraduate degree.

One of my closest university friends (a crazy, spontaneous, highly intelligent guy) happened to move to my home city to work, where he quickly formed a new social circle. It would have been impossible for him not to. He is an absolute people magnet, and one of my favourite people ever; he also happens to be gay, rendering our brother-sister type bond even more intimate and special. I experience my friendship with him – and everything we do together – in an extremely intense way, because he has always pushed me out of my comfort zone and connected me with other unconventional, likeminded souls. Most of the time, I'd meet my friends' friends and like them but feel no real affinity with any of them – no real potential for magic. However, this guy introduced me to a countless number of fascinating people while I was at university – a few of whom definitely 'glimmered' to me, but who (luckily) weren't the precise archetype I was susceptible to falling for at that time.

I still felt painful, painful things for my first LO (LO1) at this point, but I had left university, waved goodbye to the city (where he stayed to work) and returned to my own. I'd spend at least 1/2 of my day thinking about him/craving that specific feeling he'd give me, but I was **past the 'crystallised' stage of limerence** - no longer crying my eyes out multiple times a day and wanting to die. I wasn't enjoying life, but I was living it once again.

I was also able to see flaws in his personality – he affected me emotionally, but my logical mind was luckily *no longer adamant* that he was the only one for me. I was ready to connect with someone else… to be 'drugged' by someone else and forget him.

Little did I know, that attitude of mine effectively primed me, there and then, for a second, equally derailing limerent episode; I was telling my subconscious mind "**look for intensity, chaos and sharp emotions**. When you find them in someone new, amplify them and lose yourself in them. Search for someone who triggers you emotionally, but who is, in many ways, his opposite. That's how you'll forget him."

Moreover, I was still completely failing to see that this obsessive experience – these pangs of 'love' – were revealing things about myself, and problematic elements of my own psychology (i.e. things I could actually change and improve). I knew I had to detach from him and saturate myself with things that were different to him/what he stood for, but I didn't realise that I *simultaneously* needed to *draw the line under limerence as a state* - under being the version of myself who can become limerent.

I was viewing 'love' in a highly deterministic manner, failing to grasp that these limerent feelings didn't just 'happen' to unlucky people… they were the result of a tonne of different factors. I needed to crack the root causes of my limerence problem and immunise myself against all possible future LOs. I now know that this is achieved by subconscious reprogramming, 'killing off' problematic aspects of your old self-concept and living in such a way that **no one can hijack your brain**. There are very specific ways to go about this, and I'm telling you all, they really work. This book is worth its weight in gold – please heed Lucy's advice and implement the right techniques, as they will truly *permanently* protect you from limerence.

Back to my story – back to how I fell into *another* (and my last) crippling limerent episode. I met my second LO (who I shall refer to as LO2) at a house party that my friend threw in his flat, and she instantly stood out to me as 'unique'. Now, that's saying something, as every single individual this friend had introduced me to has been highly individualistic, intelligent, passionate, and unconventional in style.

But gosh, the impact this girl had on me when I first met her. My height with jet black, wavy hair and dark brown eyes, she just **stood out as incredibly 'knowing'** – present, discerning and perceptive… radiating a level of 'awareness' that no one else in the room was quite tuning into. She wasn't beautiful, with quite roughened features; I was also not instantly attracted to her, despite having experimented with dating girls before. However, **I saw pure *authenticity*** in her and instantly knew that she would come to mean a lot to me. When our mutual friend introduced us, we looked each other in the eye and it was surreal – it felt incredibly meaningful and exciting, without being obviously romantic. This, I have since come to find, is typically how I experience initial romantic chemistry with girls. It's like the connection between myself and the rare girls I like is so, so complex, nuanced and spiritual (by virtue of us both being girls and reading each other's minds) that it *can't* be initially experienced by us in a simple, blatantly romantic way.

And just in that intense, but dreamy, way, we were drawn to each other like moths to a flame. We spent the entire night talking, and it felt like the realest connection I had ever experienced. That isn't something I say generically, but rather, it's the one word I can use to describe the feelings that washed over me. A certain **raw, undeniable authenticity** that I hadn't felt with my LO1 seemed to underlie the connection. I was madly in love with him and all that he represented, but I guess I never felt completely 'read' by him in the moment... like he was truly seeing me for who I was, *there and then*, wherever we were.

This didn't matter to me at the time – it was just a different bond. We did, obviously, had an incredibly deep connection and were aligned in a meaningful way. But, I guess what I'm saying is that it was always more about the 'distant, idyllic dream world' that he opened up for me. The world in which we'd both be the most accomplished, well-rounded, confident forms of ourselves. The world I always felt us moving towards, together.

You see, LO1 and I always connected on the basis of our shared dreams, shared pride and shared perfectionism... our shared love for beautiful, well-executed outcomes, for growth, for momentum. **That was it,** *momentum* – with LO1, I felt a very tangible sensation of progressing forward, together. With this girl, however, it felt like **time stopped altogether**. Chalk and cheese, two entirely different romantic states. Truly mind-blowing to be capable of experiencing both... and to end up so damaged by both.

You can probably guess where this is going – unlike my connection with my first LO (who I at least dated initially), the palpable 'spark' that this girl (LO2) and I felt was never taken to its logical endpoint. In other words, we never even kissed, let alone lived out a romantic relationship.

I rapidly discovered that **she had a long-term girlfriend**, a girl she was clearly fond of but no longer intrigued or moved by. I say this so confidently because LO2 had a lot of energy to share with others, but poured precisely zero of it towards this girlfriend of hers. She'd come to some of the parties I'd see LO2 at, but they never acted like a couple, always spending most of the night apart and speaking to different people. Her girlfriend was bold, unconventional and blunt like her – too much like her. I saw it clear as day, even though it was far from being my business... that was the problem.

There was **no polarity in their relationship**, which was why they were a poor match. There was no true 'masculine vs feminine' balance, which I believe is what differentiates love from platonic friendship, even in same-sex relationships. It doesn't matter if a lesbian couple consists of two very physically feminine women, or if one is more masculine-presenting… *mentally*, at least a few of their traits need to be functional opposites. Without this polarity, passion fizzles out, and the emotional connection either morphs into a friendship or starts to ebb away altogether.

LO2, you see, is probably the girl with the most masculine mentality I've ever met. The second time we chatted, she flippantly told me that one of her favourite pastimes was playing online multiplayer games and **pretending to be a boy,** chatting to strangers with a fake name like 'Jack'… that it weirdly energised and liberated her. At this point, we had already had several deep conversations about life, sexuality and our hopes and dreams, and this rogue little comment of hers piqued my curiosity beyond belief. If any of our mutual friends had told me something similar, it would've made me laugh, but I instead felt immensely moved (!). Felt that she'd let me in on a secret of momentous weight.

It was then that it suddenly dawned on me that this peculiar girl *had an entire life* of her own – a life that often involved her ***alone in her room*** doing such things, thinking, *being*. The idea of this 'reality' of her existence, which stretched beyond our addictive and exciting interactions, thrilled me. I wanted to be a part of that life, of her *ordinary life*, in a serious way; I wanted to know exactly what her thought processes were like, what she'd write in a diary, how she, personally, made sense of the mundanities of life. What she woke up and thought about – how she drank her coffee, and whether it gave her a buzz like it did me.

My growing interest in her life didn't settle at mere nosiness. I also wanted *her* to know that **she could text me** whenever she felt the superficial urge to 'pass as a boy'. Even if it was light-hearted entertainment to her, I wanted her life to feel so fulfilling and 'real' to her that silly pastimes like that didn't even cross her mind.

And, the truth was, I felt that the nature of our connection (i.e. the way I could make *her* feel) would probably satiate her urge to sit around at home and do such things. I could free her and take her to emotional heights far higher than her current relationship ever could, that I was sure of. Unlike her tough, feisty current girlfriend, **I would *soften* in her presence** and allow her to feel strong, protective and .. slightly 'male'… if that was what she wanted. I hate simplifying the gender roles like that, but it's the only way I can describe this girl and her unique nature: she wanted to *protect others* and be seen as strong. That was so important to her; **an unmet need of hers, for sure**. A version of herself that she couldn't access with her headstrong, combative girlfriend (who despised people 'mollycoddling' her), or with most of her friends (who were boisterous guys she joked around with, but shared no intimacy with).

However, she wasn't all masculine-leaning. She also had vulnerabilities, a girlish impishness and the tendency to be highly sentimental (telling me she cried frequently – another confession of hers that shook me to the core). Importantly, she also possessed highly developed, female-typical emotional capabilities. Her intuition was partly the reason why I was so drawn to her – because we could exchange a mere look and share worlds of information with each other, giving rise to that feeling of 'being understood and experiencing the present moment to the max' that I hadn't felt with LO1.

But, she'd always then return back to her baseline state, which was hyper-independent (despite wanting to be close to me at all times), grounded, direct and, above all, fearless. I saw all of her facets and just wanted to **allow her to be her beautiful self**: a unique mix of masculine and feminine that I had not quite seen before, and which unlocked so much joy and magic in me.

Despite me being driven, my natural state is curious, warm and free-flowing; I cringe as I type it, but I'll go ahead and say that I 'channel feminine energy' when I'm content and relaxed. This gave rise to a wonderful polarity between us, allowing her to feel captivated by me – I quite literally 'unlocked' behaviour in her that I doubt her own girlfriend ever did. It was obvious that I impacted her a tonne. ... that so much thought went into the messages she'd send me between the times that we'd see each other, that she wanted to protect me and help me achieve my dreams. She was also obviously extremely physically attracted to me, often shy to look me in the eye.

I had never had *true emotional chemistry* with a girl before, despite having casually dated a couple. She'd ask me lots of questions about my bisexuality and tease me, telling me I was 'probably really just a straight girl'. She couldn't believe I was actually bisexual, she'd say, because I looked too feminine - my hooped earrings, immaculate makeup and soft voice were apparently irreconcilable with her vision of the LGBTQ+ world. But I knew she was joking and trying to steer the conversation ever-so-subtly towards the realm of sexuality, and I loved it – it was our way of flirting. It was our way of addressing the obvious: the fact that **serendipitously meeting each other** had been the best thing to happen to both of us in months, and that she preferred me to her girlfriend. That by not dating, we were going against the grain of our carefree 'you only live once' natures – that it hurt us both a lot.

But maddeningly, we never did date or confess our feelings properly – neither of us wanted to shake things up. You see, she had got to know my close male friend (who had introduced us) and our *entire group of mutual friends* through her girlfriend... technically, she'd also met *me* through her girlfriend. She feared her a little, I could tell – feared pushing the limits or seeming suspicious. But, above all, she loathed the idea of becoming *that* girl who 'steals' all of her partner's friends and contacts (being cool, nonchalant and edgy, that so wasn't my LO2's style). But that didn't stop her talking to me exclusively any time we threw a party as a group or went on a daytrip; her girlfriend would always be chatting away to other people, anyway.

It around this time (the end of July) that that I realised how truly romantic my feelings towards this girl were becoming. My goodness, **my limerent state had *crystallised*.** It was no longer the vague realisation that she simply 'impacted me' or that I 'felt good around her', which is how it always starts: diffusely, with you half-kidding-yourself that you just 'really like the group of friends' that they're part of, or the class you're both studying. No, I *now* knew that it was very much a state that SHE was inducing in me. A girl who I certainly wasn't romantically bound to in any official way, and who I could barely even call a 'good friend'. Yet, a girl I felt more connected to than I did to anyone else.

This was when the experience took on a very tangible, and scarily 'human', quality; I say scary, because it dawned on me that **I could no longer lie to myself** – hanging out with her occasionally, and joking around, wasn't enough. I knew that I truly cared about her, and wanted to cherish her, in ways that I had never felt for a boy. Wanted to date her, and for us to live together happily ever after. To post photos on social media with her, and write her little poems. What's more, I wanted to know everything that went on in her head. I've already described this 'excessive curiosity' in-depth, but I'm bringing it back up because I want to stress just how peculiar, obsessive and downright unhealthy this component of my second limerent episode was.

Of course, all expressions of 'love' involve obsessive analysis and rumination, but with LO1, it had been purely about how he viewed me – in many ways, I considered his admirable, driven self to be somewhat static. Perfect, interesting and wonderful, sure, but relatively 'fixed' – he **represented a real, stable ideal** in my head, in the presence of which I felt *that I could also* blossom. But I never found myself wondering what precise wavelength he was on at 7am on a Thursday, or why he preferred certain songs over others. Every last thing this girl did, on the other hand, left me guessing, analysing and deducing. She just seemed so **changeable, multifaceted and *expansive*** to me. So fascinating.

Her energy seemed to bleed in all directions – even though it felt like time stopped when we were together, her presence kept permeating outwards, saturating everything. **Very psychedelic**, really – LO1, I guess, had felt like more of a clean stimulant to me (hence why I felt so much 'momentum' with him, whereas with LO2, it was about authenticity and maximally enjoying the present moment). But no, I *needed to know* everything about LO2, down to the very last thought that crossed her mind during the day, and her reasoning for doing specific things that we perhaps didn't talk about so much (like attending the gym, which she loved. Did it give her a 'rush' and help her feel strong? Or was it her inner little girl encouraging her to relax and do fun, invigorating things?).

I spent quite literally hours pondering such bizarre things.

Limerence is a crazy state; it truly *is* **goal-oriented thinking gone wrong**... channelled where it should never, ever be channelled. The motivation I felt to analyse every last thing about this girl was impressive, albeit absurd. But it felt perfectly logical during this chapter, because the goal felt worth *dying for*; as Lucy describes so well in this book, what we limerents all really want is **complete emotional enmeshment** with our LOs. I wanted this girl, her energy and her life (whether exciting or, in reality, quite boring (I didn't care!)) to consume me entirely.

This was, of course, completely **reflective of MY unmet needs and wounds** at the time... completely *unromantic*, completely my own problem, and one I ought to have rapidly addressed and got over. But, of course, what actually ensued were months of limerent delusionality, which I regrettably (and incorrectly) believed represented the 'pinnacle of my romantic life', a.k.a. true love.

It won't surprise you that these powerful new feelings caused me to completely forget about LO1. Suddenly, I felt convinced that what I'd felt for him had 'never been that big of a deal' or 'even that intense'. Oh, this is hilarious to look back on; the delusions that come along with this state, on so many different levels! In reality, I had cried every single day for the best part of a year over LO1. My mood had been entirely controlled by him, and I had prayed for my suffering to end. But, the craziest thing was that the **emotional world that *LO2* was newly providing me with** allowed the bulk of my feelings for LO1 to just vanish.

I no longer felt that I needed 'access' to the states he put me in, nor felt like I wanted to be 'that version' of myself that I felt he induced in me. So, my addiction to him (or, really, to the concept of him) started to decisively dwindle.

I barely *remembered* how it had felt to yearn for him, and for his acceptance and unconditional love. Since **limerence is so needs-based** and desperate by nature, you do rapidly heal and forget about individual LOs when those needs of yours are assuaged by something else. It's like being starving, craving a particular sandwich, but eventually eating something else and forgetting all about it – forgetting how intense and real the desire to eat it (and to be promised huge quantities of it) had been, just like that. *Laughing* at your former self for caring about one set of ingredients so much.

Upon experiencing this abrupt emotional transition, I *should've* thought "I've jumped from one person to the next in the space of twenty-four hours. Here's my proof that limerence is pathological, delusional, ridiculous, not real love, and, therefore, something to squash with a positive, future-focused mentality. So, let's focus on the root issue – the common denominator (which is *clearly me*) – and do some powerful balancing work to nip this second limerent episode in the bud."

It's weird. A part of me did realise all of the above, but the limerent emotions were so strong (and I was still so naïve) that I somehow *didn't fully believe* that it was 'just limerence' this time around. Cue the typical self-justifying limerent thoughts: 'it's different because she's a girl', '*this time it's real*', etc. – you'll all be reading this and relating, while simultaneously rolling your eyes. That's always how limerence goes: different faces, different situations, same illusory 'spiritual significance' that keeps you trapped until you actually dare to question it and obliterate it.

But, that was how I ended summer in my home city before starting my glossy new PhD programme: finally able to see that my connection with LO1 had been unwanted, unrequited limerence, but utterly convinced that my obsession with LO2 was **earth-shatteringly, agonisingly real love** that I had to hold onto.

The PhD work was stimulating and I enjoyed the course, excited to finally be on the way to calling myself Dr. But mentally, I was elsewhere, and would've given it all away for LO2. The text messages I'd sporadically receive from her represented the only real emotional sustenance I was receiving in life. They came quite often, but her energy wasn't the same as before. She was definitely still interested in me romantically, but the thing is, she clearly didn't harbour irrational feelings for me – wasn't desperate to 'lock me down' or advance our connection in brave, meaningful ways. Fair enough. She had a girlfriend, after all, and probably wasn't limerent.

But, why was she interacting with me like that, then? Why was she staying up until 4am on worknights to message me, and slipping into that specific 'state' with me – that state of **unbridled romantic curiosity**, the type that has you sending people music recommendations, asking them about their childhood, seeing **connections and synchronicities** everywhere – if she seemed simultaneously okay with seeing me occasionally and never making 'us' real? She was a smart, logical girl who spoke five languages perfectly and got whatever she wanted in life, so I couldn't quite work out how this type of half-baked, promising connection fitted into her life. Didn't she crave more than this – wasn't it obvious that we had *never been 'just friends'*?

I mean, meeting each other had obviously been incredibly euphoric for us both. Did she still feel that 'jolt' but ignore it, and repress it? if so, why? We were young, and breakups weren't a big deal; love triumphs over everything, and she could easily move on from her girlfriend and create a new life with me. Dwelling in a weird limbo state didn't seem her style. But, maybe she was just deep, intense and ready to click with likeminded people, but somehow detached in a sense… perhaps completely different to me, in ways I'd never previously contemplated…? In ways that meant she liked me a whole lot, but didn't feel obsessed or in love… at all?

Such rumination **yielded zero conclusions** and only fuelled my addiction. Nonetheless, it consumed my every waking hour. My confusion, however, was 'rational' in a sense, given my feelings; our connection (and the mixed signals she'd constantly send my way) did make no sense.

Eventually, I managed to think a little more rationally and came to a conclusion of sorts: that it <u>didn't really matter how she viewed me</u>. That the connection wasn't advancing, regardless, so I could at least conclude that she *wasn't limerent* for me. I decided that **I must be very special to her** (she'd still send me little presents and slip in overtly romantic comments now and then), but in a healthy, manageable way, perhaps? A world away from the desperate, heart-breaking feelings I harboured for her, which were akin to a baby craving attention/food/its mother. Actually, I can't even compare them to something so biologically sane – babies need to grasp for things to stay alive. I, on the other hand, had no right or real reason to viscerally crave this girl's energy and attention to the extent that I did.

Moreover, being in that ludicrous, needy state actually rendered it impossible for her to even see me as she had before… impossible for me to 'get' the fantasy outcome that I wanted. Since we were both living in the same city, what I desired most was, of course, for her to tell me that passion had driven her to break up with her girlfriend. That we'd be able to start a proper, shameless, requited life chapter together. That we'd finally be able to **make it real**, giving ourselves what I 'felt' we deserved.

149

Despite having assimilated the notion that she wasn't **madly in love with me**, I was not okay. At this point, my emotions were truly getting the better of me. The depression was unrelenting, and I'd wake up tearful, swigging down coffee in an attempt to engage my rational prefrontal cortex and power through the morning. It typically did work, but the pain would creep back in, later on in the day. My desire for complete emotional reciprocation from LO2 (including both *confirmation from her* that we were as emotionally intertwined as I felt we were and the *promise* that we'd ALWAYS remain connected) overpowered my rational mind completely.

I felt I needed her more than I needed to drink water. Funnily enough, I felt so lost in my limerent misery that it actually started to dawn on me that this **wasn't really about sexuality, attraction or *even romance***. Above all, she was an *emotional* vice. I didn't even think she was that *objectively* attractive. But, a like from her on Instagram meant more to me than the surprise 25th birthday party that my parents planned for me, and certainly more than the 90% score I received in the first conference I gave as a PhD scholar.

I'd prepared well for it and dealt with the questions quite effortlessly, but who cared? Definitely not me. Even if I had successfully cured cancer, I'm sure I would've still been eaten up by that specific, pitiful self-hatred that comes along with being limerence-prone and not yet aware of how to deal with it. Being incapable of making my own life colourful left me feeling like a complete and utter loser. And, being ceaselessly reminded of the fact that most other young adults had romance/their love lives 'under control' only made matters worse.

I'd watch other couples cheerfully and calmly file in and out of restaurants, open picnic hampers at the park and even bicker over trivial things, thinking 'see, this is romance: a normal, feasible facet of life for most people. One of *many* facets of life, not its sole focus – not a drug experience, or a rollercoaster ride. What's wrong with me – why can't my emotions be triggered by **normal, achievable romantic outcomes?**'

I felt horrendous – alienated from the world, spiteful, furious, and simply going through the motions. My patience was at an all-time-low, and I could no longer fake being happy for other couples. The obvious chip I had on my shoulder (and my bizarre preoccupation with romance/people's relationship statuses in general) didn't go unnoticed. My friends were there for me when I needed them, but it was hard for us to spend quality time together because I was exuding such noxious, wounded energy.

But, a sufficiently sentimental text from LO2 (i.e. one that reminded me of the obvious soft spot that she had for me) made everything okay again. They'd transform my mood, allowing me to once again **cut through life with ease** and a playful smile. *Dangerous, dangerous, dangerous*. I was in full-blown dependence at this point, which represents the lowest pits of any form of addiction: needing the stimulus to simply feel normal and function. Consequently, my behaviour was highly unstable, which I can now (fondly) laugh at.

I remember planning a party while feeling 'up', inviting ten of my friends over, only to sink into depression/withdrawal on the day and nearly cancel the event. But, just as I was about to fake a miserable excuse and send it to the group chat, LO2 sent me a hand-drawn iMessage of something that had 'reminded me of her', giving me a new lease of life and spurring me on to host an amazing night.

But unfortunately for me, the 'fixes' she provided me with came less and less reliably. She'd respond to me if I reached out and *did* obviously care about me, but my energy was pushing her away. And not surprisingly – **I was no longer the bright**, witty, self-assured soul she had first met and felt so drawn to. People don't like to feel that they can control you like a puppet, or like you're monitoring their every move and hoping for a certain outcome – act like that with your own parents, and you'll see even *them* pull away a little.

I noticed she was sending me fewer and fewer pictures (typically of her during the day, doing random things), and that her messages were somehow less fanciful, less elaborate, more jokey. **More *platonic* (what horror)**. She even called me 'dude' a few times, which made me feel nauseous; in hindsight, it's obvious to me that she was shifting towards viewing me in that way because I was committing the classic limerent error of *copying her style* – copying the emojis she adorned her messages with, copying her jovial, blunt, tomboyish way of joking etc. – thinking that *that way*, there would be less distance between us. That I had a chance of 'drawing her in' and getting what I wanted if I **smoothed out** 'potential tensions' between us, i.e. natural differences in our energy and communication style. That if I mirrored her, I'd get her.

What a scarcity mentality, and what flawed thinking; that is not how *any human connections*, particularly romantic ones, ever work. Polarity, contrast and mystery are crucial – existing happily as yourself, and putting your own, unique spin on whatever you do, is a prerequisite to attracting the right person. Not that she *was* 'the right person' (there is no 'one' soulmate for anyone), by the way, or that I wished I had actually dated her; in my current place of clarity, I'm delighted that we never dated. I now see just how *immature* her behaviour was, too – how happy she was to maintain an unlabelled emotional connection with me that we both knew was going nowhere.

Her behaviour really revealed **a complete lack of boundaries,** and a certain childish impulsivity: "we click well and have a special connection, but let's just flirt and have deep chats while I continue to date my girlfriend. Oh, and I'll also send you occasional presents, music and little drawings throughout the day. I'm just living in the moment, and I do like you: you're special, inquisitive and beautiful, and I want you to achieve every goal you've ever set yourself. Trust me, when I say that very few people wake up these feelings in me. But don't get it twisted – we aren't really anything. Let's not overcomplicate this or even acknowledge our obviously intimate bond."

A perplexing and complex girl, sure. An equally perplexing and complex connection. But spiritually meaningful and somehow the epitome of 'true love'? I don't think so. In reality, I was just as much to blame for how long it lasted, if not more to blame. We were both caught up in a silly, relatively *meaningless* dance.

I started to *properly* research limerence that January, keen to grasp what it meant for me. Propelled by a fiery mixture of pain, self-hatred, and the growing realisation that my feelings were neither normal nor *of any use* to me, **I committed to getting over LO2.**

When I came across Lucy's book, I had a complete and utter epiphany. I suddenly so clearly saw what was going on; before, I had dismissed the idea of my feelings being 'limerence' because it all felt so real, and she seemed too intriguing and complex to be **a generic 'LO'**. But I got over myself, quickly realising that those *very feelings of certainty* are quite literally a symptom of the condition, that everyone feels that their LO is the 'love of their life', whether it's their narcissistic boss, their friend's partner or just an acquaintance who barely gives them the time of day. And that when limerents work on themselves and recover, they always roll their eyes at their former selves, wondering why on earth this individual's name even stood out to them.

That was when I began to see her for who she really was, coming to conclusions like the ones I've skimmed over above; what my limerent mind was *perceiving* to be **'hyper-profound'** about LO2 could just as easily have been described as ***attention seeking***, non-committal, or (as I don't think she ever intended any harm) just plain immature. Most relevantly, however, it dawned on me that I had ironically *only* become limerent for LO2 because I had handled my feelings for LO1 *horrifically* – in a completely amateur way.

Unaware that I should view my feelings for LO1 as *a pure vice,* I partially romanticised them, unwilling to renounce the addiction I was stuck in and move forward – the addiction to feeling affirmed, powerful and capable alongside him. Or, more accurately, the addiction *to the delusion* that I could only be this way with his influence towering over me in life. When I arrived back in my home city the summer after my undergraduate degree, I was subconsciously *and* consciously **desperate to fall for someone else**. I believed that potent feelings/pain could only be replaced by *similar, even more potent* feelings/pain.

Naturally, I quickly clicked with and fell for someone more intuitive, more emotional, and more mysterious than LO1 – more crazy and carefree. Because I had, in a sense, overcome the unmet needs that had initially allowed me to become so obsessed with him: I was no longer desperate for someone to be my mentor, for a powerfully perfectionistic, stoic partner. But, I had replaced them with new 'unmet needs', or let new ones manifest in my character. These are precisely what allowed LO2 to 'glimmer' to me; suddenly, I needed intensity, playfulness, to **live the present moment in a unique, psychedelic way** that took me far away from my world of academics and perfectionism (which I associated with him at the time).

Of course, what I really ought to have done was balance different sides of my personality, strengthen my foundations and **build myself back up from scratch** - I needed to become a version of myself who <u>wasn't walking around with any</u> huge, infinitely deep unmet needs. Who wasn't aching for affirmation from others and constant enmeshment – who wouldn't fall head-over-heels for blurry, immature romantic connections that were reminiscent of the crushes most people have (and get tired of) around age sixteen.

Because LO2 and I never even came close to dating – never had a proper date, never spoke *completely* honestly about how much we meant to each other, and certainly wouldn't have worked out. The connection would never have been as magical as I had imagined, had we been able to live together as girlfriends; limerence lies to you.

And, just like that, I suddenly saw it all so clearly. It was me, and my psychological issues, that had actively aligned me with the strange, unconventional dynamic that I shared with LO2, making it seem alluring, poignant and incredibly significant. When it was really half-baked, insincere and silly.

Be very careful – your brain, by default, is designed to make <u>whatever it thinks will 'help you survive'</u> seem special, sacred and important in this way. Depending on who you are, this might mean limerence, or an addiction to alcohol/exercise/whatever. Fortunately, **you always have the power** to rapidly transform yourself into someone who can no longer be affected *in that way* by the stimulus in the first place. Who can't become addicted again, can't reach the lows again, can't be derailed again. Work out what's behind this limerence problem of yours and do the self-work – you will be blown away by how rapidly you overcome it.

I'm delighted that I'm now free, and grateful to have received LO2 as a catalyst to learn how to actually beat limerence.

It's ironic; the condition's all about trying to become 'one' with someone, but it inspires you to do the very things that actually render a real, normal connection with them impossible. Yet, when you dare to take the leap, do the correct self-work and shift your mentality, you're always *delighted that you never* did end up in a requited relationship with your LO. That you were brave enough to distance yourself from your emotions, figure out what they were screaming at you, conceptualise the situation differently, and learn from it. If you are reading this and in a **state of deep limerence**, there's one thing I can promise you – limerence is the best opportunity for self-improvement that will ever come your way, so grab it and fly with it. Show yourself what you're capable of.

Afterword

I hope you have found these individuals' raw, candid, incredibly brave depictions of limerence to be of value. That you'll be able to identify with some of the **uniquely limerent** doubts, thought loops and emotions that they've described, and learn from their revelations. And that the stories that are *dissimilar* to your own will help you nonetheless, by providing you with the highly comforting evidence that limerence is completely treatable, regardless of how it manifests itself. That it is a bizarre, destructive state involving unbridled emotions and delusionality, but that it is also, at the end of the day, a **human issue**. One whose outward appearance can vary as much as we can, but which is, like us, fairly homogeneous on the inside. And that for this reason, we can treat it with the same, relatively simple toolbox.

Above all, I hope you are now able to see your personal limerence pattern for *what it is:* something that you are genetically prone to, for sure, but something that **you are now equipped** to protect yourself from for the rest of your life. Something that you can rapidly shift yourself out of, by honouring who you really are, saturating yourself with exciting energy and fulfilling things, and setting yourself new, inspiring goals. The overarching prerequisite to recovery being, of course, that you align with a new, limerence-immune version of yourself by altering your subconscious wirings.

Sometimes, when we first wake up to the truth about limerence and realise that we must take matters into our own hands and recover, we go about it the wrong way: by forcing ourselves to proactively move through life while 'distracting ourselves'. Occasionally, this '**stoic**

autopilot state' will be essential during the earliest stages of recovery; you will, at times, feel despondent, yet still have to take care of an array of different responsibilities.

However, this 'power through it' phase will be over before you know it, as long as you adhere to the recovery techniques and maintain a future-focused attitude. As you will now realise, the **primary goal in recovery** is always to speak to your subconscious mind. This is what alters who you are on a fundamental level (and, by virtue, how external stimuli can make you feel in the first place). Through additionally honouring your psychological needs, connecting with new people who enrich your life in healthy, unique ways, learning to celebrate your nature as it is, giving yourself room to grow and challenging yourself, you will not even *need to think* about being 'sensible'. You will no longer have to handle that horrible, gnawing pain you are so familiar with, for it will be absent. You will have effectively **transmuted it** into higher states of consciousness: clarity, emotional coherence and contentedness.

Nor will you have to 'avoid triggering people' or worry about 'potential LOs'. There ***will be no* triggers** capable of sending you into artificial states of utter delusionality like limerence, for you will be living in consonance with who you really are. You will feel inspired, playful and balanced, and will react to the world in a congruent manner. This will automatically render you a match for healthy, sustainable bliss, and *meaningfully* enlivening connections that bloom to their fullest, most authentic expressions and bring out the best in you. It goes without saying that limerence does not exist in such a reality paradigm, for it simply cannot.

① Initial analysis

Decide to view this as 'pathological love'.

Work out under *what* circumstances you become limerent, your **'trigger archetype'**, and *what* about these LOs makes you **feel so high** in the first place.

② Deep, introspective reflection

Commit to viewing the dynamics of your limerent connection/s *completely* objectively.

How are they *actually* treating you? (Don't make vilifying their behaviour your focus, but do get clear on what's really going on, as this will reveal **your unmet needs**). What are you **letting them represent?**

③ Meet your psychological needs & *bathe in* new feelings

Now that the causal factors behind your limerence problem are evident, prioritise meeting your needs in whatever ways you can to *free yourself from them*. This will involve you making changes in your life, which may be big (changing career, cutting off draining people) or small (allowing yourself to have deeper conversations with existing friends).

④ Construct a new self-concept with a whole new set of exciting desires/goals

Once you're actively meeting your unmet needs as much as you can, you should jump into all of the **subconscious reprogramming techniques** we covered in Chapter 28. You'll be well-poised to see rapid, magical results. In generating new beliefs about yourself/the world and setting new intentions, you'll be stepping into a new, far superior version of yourself. One that's congruent with your dream life, and incompatible with (and immune to) limerence. Persevere in it and *think from it*, until it hardens into your daily reality.

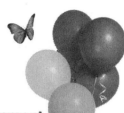

(5)   **Enjoy freedom, stability and alignment**

Congratulations; you've now achieved something of enormous significance.

You've not only overcome limerence (one of the most convincing, derailing illusions out there), but have also learnt to **live and** *thrive* **as your** *truest self*. Immune from artifice, unnecessary pain and addiction - and aligned with bliss and fulfilment.

Few people receive the wake-up call required to catalyse this type of self-transformation; consider your limerent past a ***blessing in disguise***.

As well as knowing how to skilfully channel your obsessive nature to your advantage, you now **have faith** in your ability to tackle anything - to transform any seemingly 'intractable' psychological state or situation. Which is highly, highly rare, and is something that no one can take away from you.

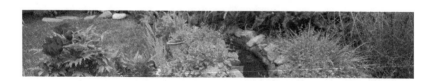

References

Here you have the resources that have aided the production of this book. I've also slipped in some extra material, for those of you interested in the world of neuroscience and/or inspired to do some further reading on all things related to limerence.

Websites:

www.neuroscientificallychallenged.com: engaging, broken-down neurobiology (a great place to start if you want to learn about neuroscience/neuroanatomy in a methodical way, and further explore the roles of the brain regions we have looked at).

www.neurosparkle.com: my own website, which I greatly enjoy posting to. I have designed it to be a safe, interesting place for pre- , mid- or post-recovery limerents who desire to reach the highest level of self-understanding possible (as well as, of course, to permanently recover from the behavioural pattern). Head over and leave a comment updating me on your recovery progress – I would love to hear from you there. Also be sure to sign up for **exclusive content and *surprises*.**

go.drugbank.com: beautiful pharmacology website that hosts information on the pharmacodynamics/kinetics of all medications under the sun. If you are interested in neuroscience and the molecular basis of mood disorders/psychiatric diseases, you'll enjoy browsing it. If you have ever taken psychiatric medication, I recommend that you do.

www.livingwithlimerence.com: a fantastic blog about limerence run by fellow neuroscientist Dr. L.

Books:

Descartes' Error by Antonio Damasio

Molecules of Emotion – Why You Feel The Way You Feel by Candace B. Pert

Incognito – The Secret Life of the Brain by David Eagleman

Thinking In Systems: A Primer by Donatella Meadows (highly recommended; it is guaranteed to sharpen your ability to conceptualise systems (including mathematical systems, the thermostat-driven heating system in your home, ecosystems, businesses, your family unit, and even yourself/your goals). If you can start to view yourself as a tweakable 'system' and your behaviour as the output, this will enable you to more effectively and rapidly a). detach from your emotions and b). take action to remedy them. It is also invaluable to understand how systems work in this day and age and some of the laws that they are all subject to (and the paradoxical phenomena that can arise under certain circumstances) – they are at the crux of so many different fields!

The Game of Life and How to Play It by Florence Scovell Schinn (the affirmation 'evil leaves no mark' was inspired by this woman's work; if it resonates with or comforts you, you will greatly enjoy her book and its many spiritual, philosophical and moral insights. Florence Scovell Schinn is, along with Joseph Murphy and Neville Goddard, one of the most influential early teachers of what is now widely described as The Law of Assumption/Belief. While the Law of Attraction depicts your desires to be far away from you, with you needing to change your energy field to 'attract' them towards you, the Law of Assumption/Belief more accurately frames the beliefs that you implant into your subconscious mind as the source of all of your joy and afflictions. While her writing is imbued with some biblical references, being Christian (or religious) is in no way a prerequisite to enjoying and learning from this book; it comprises many beautiful, highly unique affirmations/ideas to feed your subconscious).

The Power of Your Subconscious Mind by Joseph Murphy (this is a book that every one of you should get your hands on if you have had your interest piqued by the subconscious mind reprogramming techniques we have studied. Your subconscious mind influences everything from autonomic bodily processes to your daily mood, your energy levels and the thoughts and feelings that you have about the people in your life. The importance of mastery over your subconscious mind is not only wholly reconcilable with neuroscience, but is also actively endorsed by it once you dig deep, think critically and consider the brain-body connection holistically. This topic can surpass 'logical science' and dip into the realm of the surreal and numinous if you are open to esoteric things, but it equally does not need to. POSM is highly accessible regardless of your personal stances towards spirituality).

How Emotions Are Made by Lisa Feldman Barrett (also a must-read; no scientist conceptualises human emotion quite like Lisa Barrett does... her theory is daring, controversial, but undeniably, enlightening. Even if you question some of her conclusions, your ability to a). consider what emotions actually are/serve to do and b). manage your own emotions will be forever sharpened following this book).

Why We Sleep by Matthew Walker (not directly related to limerence per se, but of utmost relevance to your mood and overall wellbeing).

Feeling Is The Secret by Neville Goddard (slightly esoteric and written in a poetic manner, but highly recommended if you are a lover of science/logic but also open to having your mind pushed in other directions. Neville Goddard was a New Age teacher and author who realised the immense power that his imagination had in directing him towards specific desired 'end goals'. His techniques are life-changing and, as with those of Joseph Murphy, can either be interpreted as spiritual truths about this reality or simply moulded to fit and work with your own personal views).

The Brain That Changes Itself by Robert Doige

Behave by Robert Sapolsky (absolutely phenomenal introduction to behavioural neuroscience, from a robust biological perspective that takes into consideration anatomy, evolution, etc. If you ever to desire to read a book about human behaviour, make sure it is this one. I also recommend that you take a look at some of Prof. Sapolsky's interviews and lectures – he exudes passion for his subject and is a truly gifted science communicator).

Scientific Textbooks:

Byrne, J. and Roberts, J., 2004. *From molecules to networks*. Amsterdam: Elsevier Academic Press.

Neve, K., 2010. *The Dopamine Receptors*. Totowa, NJ: Humana Press, a part of Springer Science & Business Media, LLC.

Stone, T., 1997. *Neuropharmacology*. Oxford: Oxford University Press.

Vahia, V., 2017. *Diagnostic and statistical manual of mental disorders*. Arlington, VA: American Psychiatric Association.

Whitaker-Azmitia, P. and Peroutka, S., 1990. *The neuropharmacology of serotonin*. New York: The New York Academy of Sciences.

Scientific Publications:

Bello, N. T., & Hajnal, A. (2010). Dopamine and binge eating behaviors. *Pharmacology Biochemistry and Behavior*.

Burunat, E., 2019. Love is a physiological motivation (like hunger, thirst, sleep or sex). *Medical Hypotheses*, 129, p.109225.

Charney, D. S. (1989). The Yale-Brown Obsessive Compulsive Scale: II. Validity. *Archives of General Psychiatry*.

Earp, B., Wudarczyk, O., Foddy, B. and Savulescu, J., 2017. Addicted to Love: What Is Love Addiction and When Should It Be Treated?. *Philosophy, Psychiatry, & Psychology*, 24(1), pp.77-92.

Fisher, H., Xu, X., Aron, A. and Brown, L., 2016. Intense, Passionate, Romantic Love: A Natural Addiction? How the Fields That Investigate Romance and Substance Abuse Can Inform Each Other. *Frontiers in Psychology*, 7.

Försterling, F., & Binser, M. J. (2002). Depression, school performance, and the veridicality of perceived grades and causal attributions. *Personality and Social Psychology Bulletin*.

Goodman, W. K., Price, L. H., Rasmussen, S. A., Mazure, C., Delgado, P., Heninger, G.R.& Gorwood, P. (2004). Eating Disorders, Serotonin Transporter Polymorphisms and Potential Treatment Response. *American Journal of PharmacoGenomics.*

Hinvest, N. S., Elliott, R., McKie, S., & Anderson, I. M. (2011). Neural correlates of choice behavior related to impulsivity and venturesomeness. *Neuropsychologia.*

Jiang, Y., Kim, S. and Bong, M., 2014. Effects of reward contingencies on brain activation during feedback processing. *Frontiers in Human Neuroscience*, 8.

Leviel, V. (2011). Dopamine release mediated by the dopamine transporter, facts and consequences. *Journal of Neurochemistry.*

Rajkumar, R., Pandey, D. K., Mahesh, R., & Radha, R. (2009). 1-(m-Chlorophenyl)piperazine induces depressogenic-like behaviour in rodents by stimulating the neuronal 5-HT2A receptors: Proposal of a modified rodent antidepressant assay. *European Journal of Pharmacology.*

Startup, H., Lavender, A., Oldershaw, A., Stott, R., Tchanturia, K., Treasure, J., & Schmidt, U. (2013). Worry and rumination in anorexia nervosa. *Behavioural and Cognitive Psychotherapy.*

Schilman, E. A., Klavir, O., Winter, C., Sohr, R., & Joel, D. (2010). The role of the striatum in compulsive behavior in intact and orbitofrontal-cortex-lesioned rats: Possible involvement of the serotonergic system. *Neuropsychopharmacology.*

Simmler, L. D., Rickli, A., Schramm, Y., Hoener, M. C., & Liechti, M. E. (2014). Pharmacological profiles of aminoindanes, piperazines, and pipradrol derivatives. *Biochemical Pharmacology.*

Made in the USA
Middletown, DE
28 November 2021

53607248R00097